The Inpatient Medicine Handbook

Masahiro J Morikawa

The Inpatient Medicine Handbook

A Concise, Visual Guide to Clinical Decision-Making

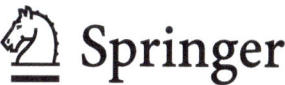

Masahiro J Morikawa
Department of Family Medicine, University of Virginia
Charlottesville, VA, USA

ISBN 978-3-032-08397-5   ISBN 978-3-032-08398-2   (eBook)
https://doi.org/10.1007/978-3-032-08398-2

This Springer imprint is published by the registered company Springer Nature Switzerland AG
The registered company address is: Gewerbestrasse 11, 6330 Cham, Switzerland

If disposing of this product, please recycle the paper.

You can only fight the way you practice

—Musashi Miyamoto

Preface

This is the 12th edition of the handbook I started in 2006. The primary motivation came from several years of my frustrating experiences as an inpatient teaching attending: How can I provide meaningful teaching without compromising a quality of patient care? How can I help residents retain essential knowledge and skills in inpatient medicine if they rotate my service only for several months a year?

Your life as a resident is unbelievably busy. The minute you walk into the hospital, your pager goes off without a break. The amount of orders and clicks you have to put in each day is astronomical, while you have to learn something practical and meaningful every single day. One thing for sure at the end of this nonstop complex problem-solving sequence and constant challenge in prioritization, that is called residency, you have to demonstrate your competency and confidence to pass the board exam.

This handbook is to rectify part of my dilemma between service and teaching as a bedside educator. I have been constantly challenging you with practical patient care questions and direct my answers to the handbook. I want you to read and enjoy as many elegant and valuable articles and monographs cited in the handbook.

This handbook is organized into four parts: fundamental topics are essential basic knowledge regardless of your specialty; several surgical topics are put together in Part II to help managing surgical patients; Part III, Essential topics are the most common problems encountered in inpatient medicine; and the handbook ends with Part IV, essential formula that you cannot forget as long as you attend sick patients. Fundamentals provide a set of vocabularies in inpatient medicine. Without sufficient vocabularies, you cannot carry out meaningful discussions with other specialists or colleagues. These fundamentals should be inculcated through your daily rounds.

The purpose of this handbook is by no means to replace standard well-circulated manuals. Rather, it is to help you better understand those existing references to gain some practical knowledge. Please remember, no patient comes with the same problems or with only one problem at a time. You have to deal with infinite combination of problems in your daily practice with whatever the knowledge and skills you have.

The references are graded by ☺ system. ☺☺☺ are the most important for everyone, ☺ would be the one you're really interested in the topic.

I believe the saying, "practice makes perfect." It is the practice that help us build our consistency and confidence in our services in any circumstances. That is a quintessential part of professionalism. Through practice, we become who we are as healers. It is we, not guidelines or protocols, who treat and heal our patients. Please enjoy.

Charlottesville, VA, USA   Mori J. Morikawa
June 2025

MORIism: Get In the Moment (GIM) Approach

They say the gate to heaven only opens if you fully get in the moment.

1. Leave your textbooks behind, get in the moment: engage and dig in.
2. Patient care is a dynamic process; Timing is crucial, and find right timing and right moment in anything you do to patients.
3. Making diagnoses is not the goal; Treatment is.
4. Your commitment, rather than pills and injections, is the treatment.
5. If you are not convinced, that treatment doesn't work on your patients.
6. You are NOT treating YOU or YOUR FEELINGS.
7. When you start treating numbers, you are not treating patients anymore.
8. Not your smartphone, but you use all what you get to see patients; your knowledge, your senses, hunch, and imagination.
9. Confidence only comes with engaging patients day in and out.
10. How hard and crazy your shift is, the end will sure to come: Get in this moment now.

It will take for a while until you understand the above. Go with your own pace.

Contents

Part I

Fundamentals

Acid-Base Interpretation

1

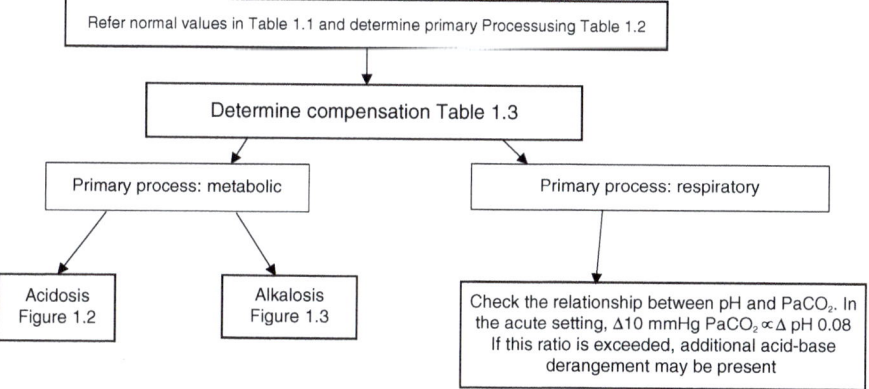

Fig. 1.1 Stepwise approach

Table 1.1   Normal values

	Normal value	Reference range
pH	7.4	7.38–7.42
$PaCO_2$	40 mmHg	38–42 mmHg
$PvCO_2$	$PVCO_2 = PaCO_2 + 6$ mmHg	≤48 mmHg
HCO_3^-	24 mEq/L	22–26 mEq/L
Anion gap (AG) = Na − (Cl + HCO_3)	<12 mEq/L	8–14 mEq/L
Calculated Osm = 2 × Na + glucose/18 + BUN/2.8	285 mOsm/L	280–295 mOsm/L
Osmolal gap (Osm gap) = measured − calculated osmolality	<10 mOsm/L	10 ± 6 mOsm/L
Urine anion gap (UAG) = Una + Uk − Ucl	<0 mEq/L	0 ± 10 mEq/L

Based on Berend et al. [1]; Palmer [2]; Martin [3]

Table 1.2   Determination of primary process

pH (reference value of 7.40)	$PaCO_2$ (reference value of 40 mmHg)	Primary process
↓	↓	Metabolic acidosis
↑	↑	Metabolic alkalosis
↓	↑	Respiratory acidosis
↑	↓	Respiratory alkalosis

Based on Narins and Emmett [4]; Palmer [2]

Table 1.3   Compensation rules

Primary acid-base disorder	Expected compensation
Metabolic acidosis	$PaCO_2 = HCO_3 + 15$
Metabolic alkalosis	$PaCO_2 = 40 + [0.7 \times (HCO_3 - 24)]$
Respiratory acidosis	$HCO_3 = 24 + [1 \times (PaCO_2 - 40)/10]$ (acute)
	$HCO_3 = 24 + [3.5 \times (PaCO_2 - 40)/10]$ (chronic)
Respiratory alkalosis	$HCO_3 = 24 - [2 \times (40 - PaCO_2)/10]$ (acute)
	$HCO_3 = 24 - [5 \times (40 - PaCO_2)/10]$ (chronic)

Based on Achanti and Szerlip [5]; Kamel and Halperin [6]
HCO_3 = bicarbonate; $PaCO_2$ = partial pressure of carbon dioxide

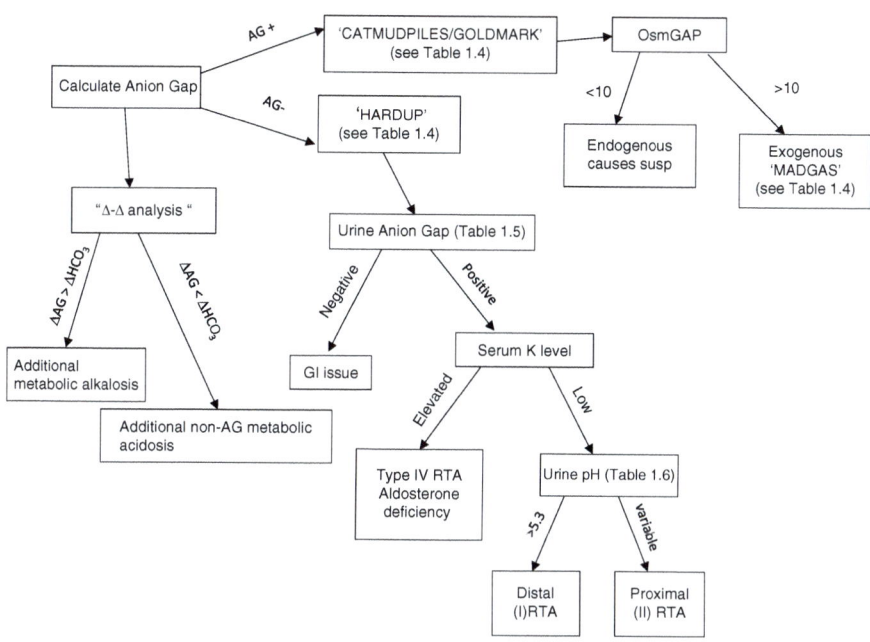

Fig. 1.2 Workup algorithm for Metabolic acidosis. Acid-base interpretation algorithm [1, 2, 7, 8]

Table 1.4 Acronym for acidosis

CATMADPILES	C: carbon monoxide	Reddy and Mooradian [9]
	A: alcohol, AKA	
	T: toluene	
	M: Methanol	
	U: uremia	
	D: DKA	
	P: paraldehyde, glycol	
	I: INH, Iron, isopropyl alcohol	
	L: lactic acidosis	
	E: Ethylene glycol	
	S: salicylates	
GOLDMARK	G: glycols (ethylene and propylene)	Mehta et al. [10]
	O: Oxoproline	
	L: L-lactate	
	D: D-lactate	
	M: Methanol	
	A: Aspirin	
	R: Renal failure	
	K: Ketoacidosis	

(Continued)

Table 1.4 (continued)

MADGAS	M: Mannitol A: alcohols D: Diatrizoate G: glycerol A: acetone S: sorbitol	Judge [11]
HARDUP	H: Hyperalimentation A: Acetazolamide R: RTA and renal insufficiency D: Diarrhea and diuretics U: Ureteroenterostomy P: Pancreatitic fistula	Casaletto [12]

Low or negative AG

- Caused by decrease in unmeasured anion or increase in unmeasured cation (hypercholoremia: lithim monocloncal IgG, Ca, Mg) [1, 13]

$\Delta - \Delta$ ($\Delta AG/\Delta HCO_3$) [14]

- Mixed disturbances should be considered if $\Delta AG/\Delta HCO_3$ <0.8 or >1.2
- If $\Delta AG/\Delta HCO_3$ <1—HCMA or respiratory alkalosis
- If $\Delta AG/\Delta HCO_3$ >1—metabolic alkalosis or respiratory acidosis

Urine anion gap (urine AG)

- Newer evidence supports measuring urine NH4, instead of UAG [15]

Table 1.5 Urine AG

UAG = (UNa + UK) − UCl	
Urine AG	Dx
Negative	Normal GI loss
Positive	Renal causes RTA Aldosterone deficiency

Based on Batlle et al. [16]

Table 1.6 RTA: urine pH and serum K

	Normal	Proximal (II) RTA	Distal (I) RTA	Type IV RTA
Urine pH	< 5.2	Variable, early stage >7.0 Late stage <5.2	>5.5	<5.2
Serum K	Normal	↓	↓	↑

Based on Soleimani and Rastegar [8]

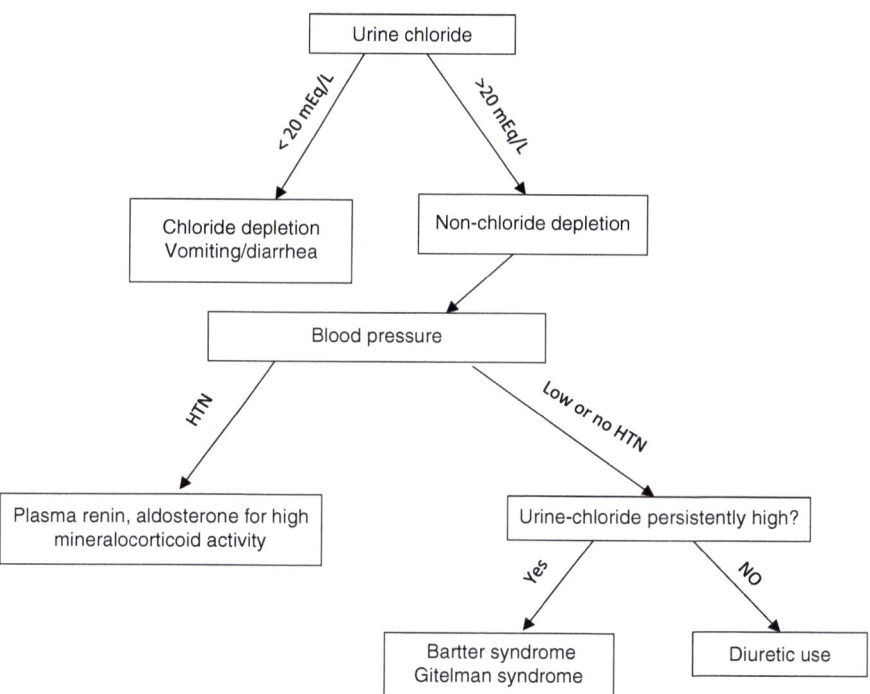

Fig. 1.3 Metabolic alkalosis. (Based on Gennari [17]; Kraut and Madias [18]; Rastegar and Nagami [19]; Kamel and Halperin [6])

Bicarb requirement in CKD

- (Desired bicarb – serum bicarb) × 50% BW (kg) [20]

How to start Bicarb?

- $NaHCO_3$ dose should be reduced if bicarb >26 mEq/L
- With sodium bicarbonate tablet, conversion of HCO_3 to CO_2 causes upper GI symptoms.
- In tablets with citric acid, conversion of citrate to HCO_3 impaired in liver disease [21].

Table 1.7 Use of bicarb for CKD

HCO_3^-	≤18 mEq/L	19–21 mEq/L
Starting dose of $NaHCO_3$	1300 mg BID	650 mg BID
Titration	Target HCO_3^- 24–26 mEq/L Titrate up to 3900 mg/day If persistently <22 mEq/L Titrate up to 5850 mg/day	

Based on Raphael [22]

References

1. ☺☺☺Berend K, et al. Physiological approach to assessment of acid-base disturbances. N Engl J Med. 2014;371:1434–45.
2. ☺☺☺Palmer B. Approach to fluid and electrolyte disorders and acid-base problems. Prim Care Clin Off Pract. 2008;35:195–213.
3. Martin, L. (1999). Primary and mixed acid-base disorders. All you really need to know to interpret arterial blood gases. Philadelphia, Lippincott Williams & Wilkins: 137.
4. Narins R, Emmett M. Simple and mixed acid-base disorders: a practical approach. Medicine (Baltimore). 1980;59(3):161–87.
5. ☺☺Achanti A, Szerlip H. Acid-base disordders in the critically ill patient. Clin J Am Soc Nephrol. 2023;18(1):102–12.
6. Kamel K, Halperin M. Fluid, electrolyte, and acid-base physiology. Philadelphia: Elsevier; 2017.
7. Whittier W, Rutecki G. Primer on clinical acid-base problem solving. Dis Mon. 2004;50:117–62.
8. ☺Soleimani M, Rastegar A. Pathophysiology of renal tubular acidosis: Core curriculum 2016. Am J Kidney Dis. 2016;68(3):488–98.
9. ☺☺Reddy P, Mooradian A. Clinical utility of anion gap in deciphering acid-base disorders. Int J Clin Pract. 2009;63(10):1516–25.
10. Mehta A, et al. GOLD MARK: an anion gap mnemonic for the 21st century. Lancet. 2008;372:892.
11. Judge B. Differentiating the causes of metabolic acidosis in the poisoned patient. Clin Lab Med. 2006;26:31–48.
12. Casaletto J. Differential diagnosis of metabolic acidosis. Emerg Med Clin North Am. 2005;23:771–87.

13. ☺Emmett M. Approach to the patient with a negative anion gap. Am J Kidney Dis. 2016;67(1):143–50.
14. ☺ ☺Rastegar A. Use of the AG/HCO3 ratio in the diagnosis of mixed acid-base disorders. J Am Soc Nephrol. 2007;18:2429–31.
15. Uribarri J, et al. Beyond the urine anion gap: in support of the direct measurement of urinary ammonium. Am J Kidney Dis. 2022;80(5):667–76.
16. ☺Batlle D, et al. The use of the urinary anion gap in the diagnosis of hyperchloremic metabolic acidosis. N Engl J Med. 1988;318:594–9.
17. Gennari F. Pathophysiology of metabolic alkalosis: a new classification based on the centrality of stimulated collecting duct ion transport. Am J Kidney Dis. 2011;58(4):626–36.
18. ☺ ☺ ☺Kraut J, Madias N. Differential diagnosis of nongap metabolic acidosis: value of a systemic approach. Clin J Am Soc Nephrol. 2012;7:671–9.
19. ☺ ☺Rastegar M, Nagami G. Non-anion gap metabolic acidosis: a clinical approach to evaluation. Am J Kidney Dis. 2017;69(2):296–301.
20. Kraut J, Madias N. Metabolic acidosis of CKD: an update. Am J Kidney Dis. 2016;67:307–17.
21. Raphael K. Metabolic acidosis in CKD: core curriculum 2019. Am J Kidney Dis. 2019;74:263–75.
22. Raphael K. Approach to the treatment of chronic metabolic acidosis in CKD. Am J Kidney Dis. 2016;67(4):696–702.

Pulmonary Gas Exchange/Pulmonary Edema/ARDS

2

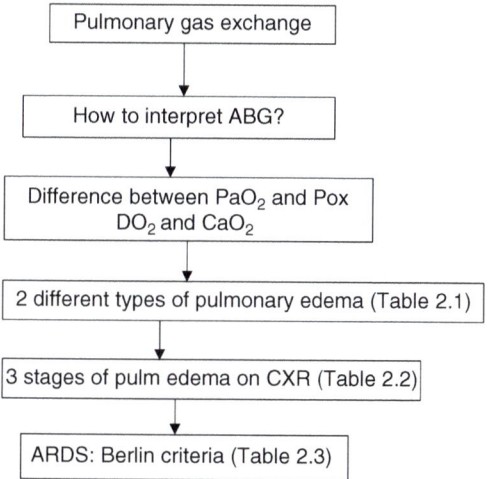

In ABG, you get following information in this order;

$$pH \,/\, PaCO_2 \,/\, PaO_2 \,/\, O_2sat$$

- The first 2 parameter, pH and $PaCO_2$ will determine primary acid-base derangement
- $PaCO_2$ is a function of ventilation: Oxygenation and ventilation are different
- $PaCO_2$ affects in ventilation, oxygenation and acid-base status

© The Author(s), under exclusive license to Springer Nature Switzerland AG 2025
M. J. Morikawa, *The Inpatient Medicine Handbook*,
https://doi.org/10.1007/978-3-032-08398-2_2

$$PAO_2 = PIO_2 - 1.2(PaCO_2)$$
$$pH = 6.1 + \log HCO_3^- / 0.03(PaCO_2)$$
$$PaCO_2 = VCO_2 \times 0.863 / VA$$

VCO_2: CO_2 production
VA: alveolar ventilation = RR × (TV − Dead space volume)

- Commonly used formula for PaO_2:

$$\boxed{PaO_2(RA) = 100 - 0.3 \times \text{age}}$$

Actual formula: 109 − 0.43 × age [1].
    In tissue level:

$$\boxed{\begin{array}{l} O_2 \text{ delivery}(DO_2) = \text{Cardiac Output}(C.O.) \times CaO_2 \\ O_2 \text{ content}(CaO_2) = 1.34 \times Hb \times \%sat(Pox) + 0.003 \times PaO_2 \end{array}}$$

$$O_2 \text{ consumption}(VO_2) = C.O. \times (CaO_2 - CVO_2)$$
$$O_2 \text{ extraction}(O_2ER) = O_2 \text{ consumption}(VO_2)$$
$$/O_2 \text{ delivery}(DO_2)$$

- Usual oxygen extraction ratio is about 24–28%

Pulmonary Edema

- Two different types: cardiogenic and non-cardiogenic [2]
- Only visible at least 30% increase in lung water [2]

Table 2.1 CXR features of cardiogenic vs noncardiogenic pulmonary edema

Cardiogenic edema	Noncardiogenic edema
Increased heart size	–
Central edema	Patchy edema
Peribronchial cuffing	Air bronchogram
Fissure line	

Ware and Matthay [2]

Table 2.2 different stages of pulmonary edema on CXR

1. Cephalization, Kerley A line
2. Interstitial edema Kerley B line
3. More central, peribronchial cuffing, fissure line (Vanishing tumor)

Berlin definition of ARDS for RI [3]

- <1 week of a known clinical insult
- Bilateral opacities in CXR
- Not fluid overload or cardia failure

$$\text{Respiratory Index}\left(\text{RI}\right) = PaO_2 \, / \, FiO_2$$

Table 2.3 Berlin criteria

Mild	Moderate	Severe
200 < RI ≤ 300 with PEEP or CPAP ≥5 cmH$_2$O	100 < RI ≤ 200 with PEEP ≥5 cmH$_2$O	RI ≤100 with PEEP ≥5 cmH$_2$O

References

1. Sorbini C, et al. Arterial oxygen tension in relation to age in healthy subjects. Respiration. 1968;25:3–13.
2. ☺ ☺ ☺Ware L, Matthay M. Acute pulmonary edema. N Engl J Med. 2005;353:2788–96.
3. Ferguson N, et al. The Berlin definition of ARDS: an expanded rationale, justificaion, and supplementary material. Intensive Care Med. 2012;38:1573–82.

Dysnatremia

3

Dysnatremia Big Picture

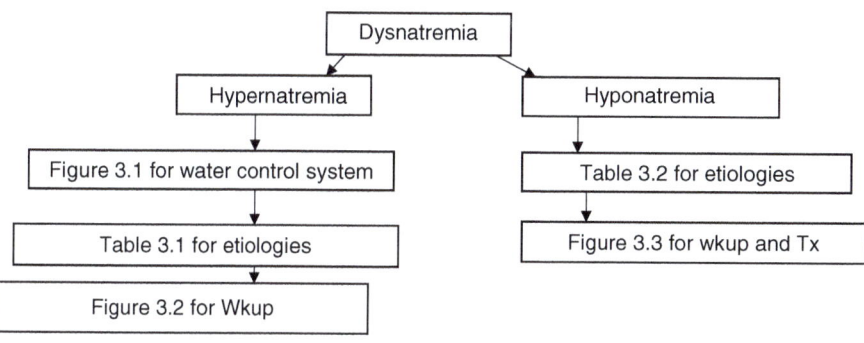

Hypernatremia

Figure 3.1 is the simple framework to sodium regulation preventing hypernatremia in our body. Table 3.1 is conceptual categorization. Figure 3.2 for flowchart for diagnosis.

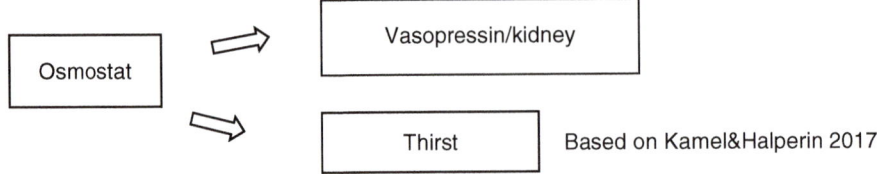

Fig. 3.1   Water control system. (Based on Kamel and Halperin [1])

Table 3.1   Etiologies of hypernatremia

	Category	Subcategory	Examples
1	Loss of water	Poor oral intake	Dementia, mental status change
		Renal loss	DI, osmotic diuresis
		GI loss	Osmotic diarrhea
		Shift	Seizure, rhabdomyolysis
2	Sodium gain	Administration	Iatrogenic IV, oral intake
		Ingestion	

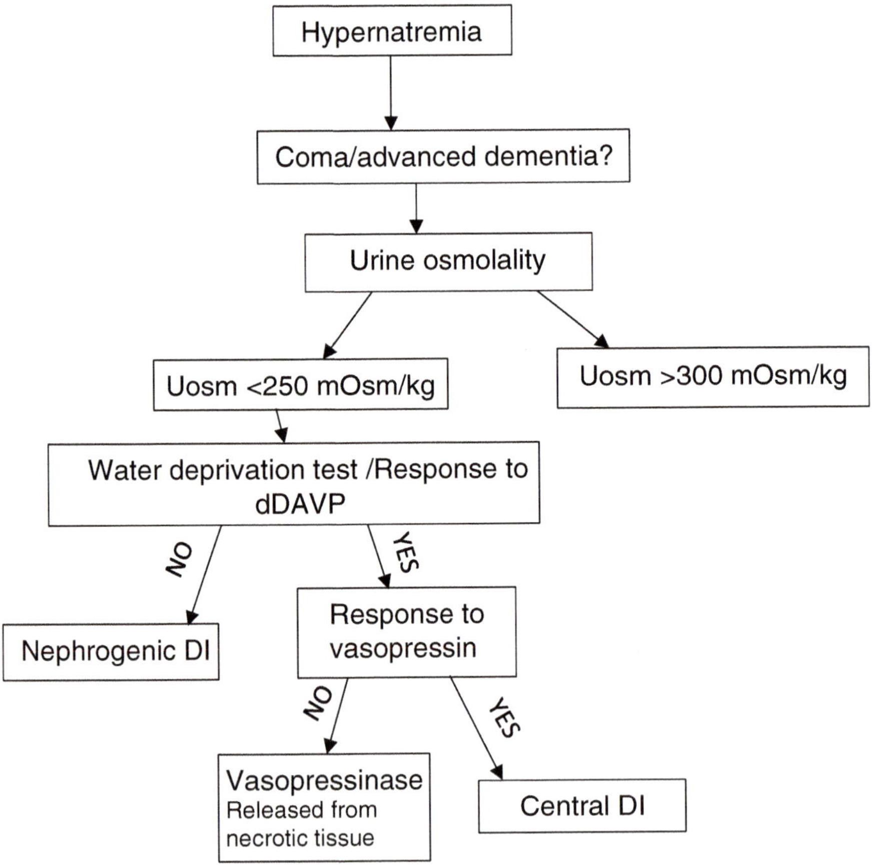

Hypernatremia

Coma/advanced dementia?

Urine osmolality

Uosm <250 mOsm/kg   Uosm >300 mOsm/kg

Water deprivation test /Response to dDAVP

NO   YES

Nephrogenic DI   Response to vasopressin

NO   YES

Vasopressinase
Released from
necrotic tissue   Central DI

Fig. 3.2   Hypernatremia wkup. (Based on Kamel and Halperin [1]; Bhasin and Velez [2])

Hyponatremia

Table 3.2 for conceptual categorization. Every hyponatremia algorithm starts with assessment of volume status, differentiating euvolemia and hypovolemia is one of the most challenging clinical judgments at the bedside. I would like to present a conceptual framework not affected by volume status except for hypervolemia which is not hard to recognize at the bedside. Figure 3.3 for simple algorithm for those without overt hypervolemia. Table 3.3 for biphasic disease. Table 3.4 for meds causing hyponatremia. Table 3.5 for DDx for SIADH and cerebral salt wasting. Table 3.6 for infusate Na contents you need to correct dysnatremia. Table 3.7 for appropriate fluid restriction strategy and Table 3.8 for predictors of failure of fluid restriction.

Table 3.2 Three categories of hyponatremia

	Na, H_2O status	ECF status	Etiology
1	Na ↑ H_2O ↑	Hypervolemic	CHF, LC, CKD
2	Na → H_2O ↑	Euvolemic	SIADH
			Psychological polydipsia
3	Na ↓ H_2O ↓	Hypovolemic	Renal loss
			GI loss
	Dilutional	–	Hyperglycemia
			Hypertriglycemia

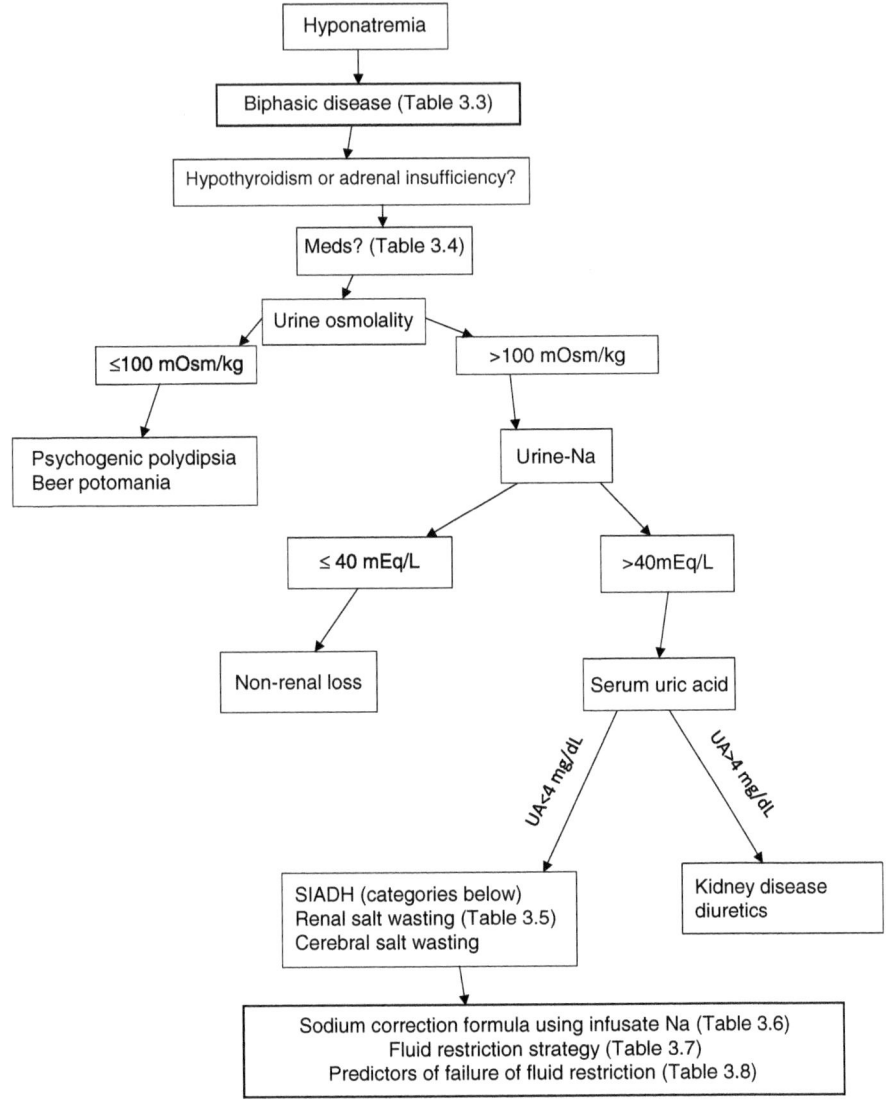

Fig. 3.3 Hyponatremia wkup. (Based on Spasovski et al. [3]; Hoorn and Zietse [4]; Adrogue et al. [5])

Symptoms

Table 3.3 Biphasic illness: hyponatremia encephalopathy and ODS

	Hyponatremic encephalopathy	ODS
Risk factors	Menstruant females Children Hypoxic patients	Chronic hyponatremia Na <105 mEq/L Hypokaleia Etoh Malnutrition Liver disease
Symptoms	HA, N/V Seizures Resp arrest Confusion	Mutism, dysarthria Dysphagia, tremor, ataxia, confusion
References	Achinger et al. [6]; Spasovski et al. [3]	Sterns et al. [13]; Verbalis et al. [7]; Laureno and Karp [8]; Abbott et al. [9]

Medications

- Citalopram is highest risk for hyponatremia among SSRI [10]

Table 3.4 Conditions and meds related to acute hyponatremia (<48 hour)

Postoperative phase
Post resection of prostate, TUR
Colonoscopy prep
Exercise (marathon)
Polydipsia
MDMA
Cyclophosphamide IV
Oxytocin
Recent HCTZ
Recent desmopressin
Recent terlipressin, vasopressin

Spasovski et al. [3]

Table 3.5 SIADH vs cerebral salt wasting

	SIADH	Cerebral salt wasting
Serum urea	Normal-low	Normal-high
Serum uric acid	Low	Low
Urine volume	Normal-low	High
Urine Na	>30 mmol/L	>>30 mmol/L
BP	normal	Normal—orthostatic hypotension
CVP	normal	Low

Spasovski et al. [3]

Four categories of SIADH [14]

1. CNS related (brain tumor, meningitis, encephalitis, SDH, EDH)
2. lung related (pneumonia, atypical pneumonia)
3. Malignancy (lung cancer, oropharyngeal cancer)
4. medications (SSRI, antiseizure medications)

Mgmt
Sodicum disorder correction formula
FORMULA: estimate the effect of infusion on correcting hyponatremia [11]
Effect of 1 L of infusion on serum Na

$$\text{Change in serum Na} = (\text{infusate Na} - \text{serum Na}) / (\text{total body water} + 1)$$

Table 3.6 Infusate Na
(mmol/L)

Infusate	Na
0.9% NS	154
LR	130
0.45% NS	77
D5 water	0

- No more than 8 mmol/L/day of change if risk for demyelination is present, if not 10–12 mEq/L/day [12]

'Rule of Sixes" [13]

- 6 mEq/L/day makes sense for safety
- 6 mEq/L in 6 hours for severe symptoms and STOP
- 4–6 mEq/L is enough correction regardless of the severity of the hyponatremia [12]

Fluid restriction

- Restrict all intake by drinking, not just water
- Aim for a fluid restriction that is 500 ml/day before the 24 hour urine volume
- Do not restrict sodium or protein intake unless indicated

Table 3.7 Strategy for fluid restriction

(Urinary Na + Urinary K)/plasma Na	Recommended fluid intake
>1	<500 ml/day
1	500–700 ml/day
<1	<1000 ml/day

Table 3.8 Predictors of failure of fluid restriction

High urine osmolality (>500 mOsm/kg H_2O)
Sum of urine Na and K exceeds the serum Na
24 hour urine volume <1500 ml/day
Increase in serum Na <2 mmol/L/day in 24–48 hours on a fluid restriction of ≤1 L/day

Based on Ellison and Berl [14]; Verbalis et al. [7]

References

1. ☺☺Kamel K, Halperin M. Use of urine electrolytes and urine osmolality in the clincial diagnosis of fluid, electrolyges, and acid-base disorders. Kidney Int Rep. 2021;6:1211–24.
2. Bhasin B, Velez J. Evaluation of polyuria: the roles of solute loading and water diuresis. Am J Kidney Dis. 2016;67(3):507–11.
3. Spasovski G, et al. Clinical practice guideline on diagnosis and treatment of hyponatremia. Intensive Care Med. 2014;40:320–31.
4. Hoorn E, Zietse R. Diagnosis and treatment of hyponatremia: compilation of the guidelines. J Am Soc Nephrol. 2017;28:1340–9.
5. ☺☺☺Adrogue H, et al. Diagnosis and management of hyponatremia. A review. JAMA. 2022;328(3):280–91.
6. ☺☺☺Achinger S, et al. Dysnatremias: why are patients still dying? South Med J. 2006;99(4):353–62.
7. ☺☺☺Verbalis J, et al. Diagnosis, evaluation, and treatment of hyponatremia: expert panel recommendations. Am J Med. 2013;126:S1–S42.
8. Laureno R, Karp B. Myelinolysis after correction of hypnatremia. Ann Intern Med. 1997;126:57–62.
9. ☺Abbott R, et al. Osmotic demyelination syndrome. BMJ. 2005;331:829–30.
10. Farmand S, et al. Differences in associations of antidepressants and hospitalization due to hyponatremia. Am J Med. 2018;131:56–63.
11. ☺☺Adrogue H, Madias N. Hyponatremia. N Engl J Med. 2000;342:1581–9.
12. ☺Sterns R. Disorders of plasma sodium- causes, consequences, and correction. N Engl J Med. 2015;372:55–65.
13. Sterns R, et al. Treating profound hyponatremia: a strategy for controlled correction. Am J Kidney Dis. 2010;56(4):774–9.
14. ☺☺☺Ellison D, Berl T. The syndrome of inappropriate antidiuresis. N Engl J Med. 2007;356:2064–72.

Dyskalemia

4

Dyskalemia Big Picture

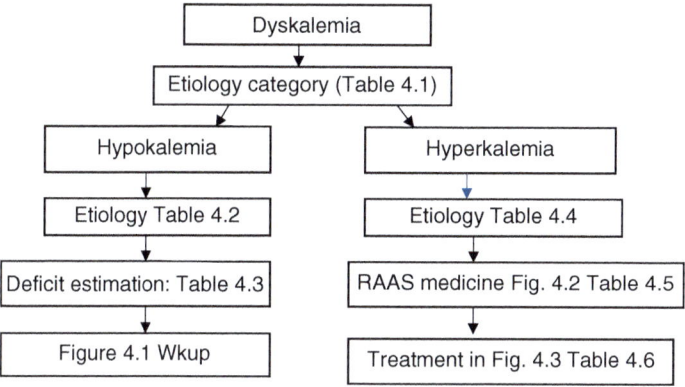

- EKG changes [1]

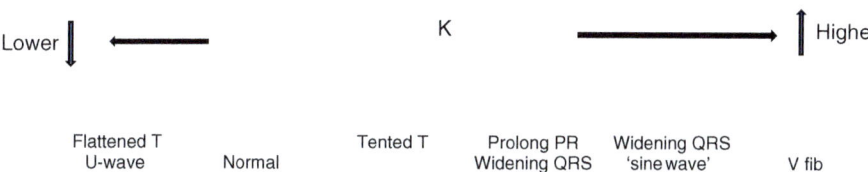

Table 4.1 Etiologies

	Hypokalemia	Hyperkalemia
1	Shift	Shift
2	Renal loss	CKD
3	Non-renal loss	Medication

Hypokalemia

Hypokalemia workup closely related to acid-base derangement please refer metabolic alkalosis algorithm in acid-base chapter. Table 4.2 shows detailed etiologies for hypokalemia. Table 4.3 for foods with high potassium, Fig. 4.1 for algorithm. Compare the algorithm with metabolic alkalosis algorithm.

Table 4.2 Causes for hypokalemia

Etiology	Examples
Shift	Metabolic alkalosis
	Beta2 agonist use
	Insulin
Renal loss	Loop, thiazide diuretics
	Osmotic diuresis
	Primary hyperaldosteronism
	Congenital adrenal hyperplasia
	Mineralocorticoid excess
	RTA
	Bartter's + Gitelman's syndrome
Non-renal loss	Diarrhea, laxative use

Gennari [1]; Palmer and Clegg [2]

Table 4.3 Deficit estimation

Estimate of potassium deficit = $(4.0 - \text{current K}) \times 100$ mEq/L

Faubel and Topf [3]

Potassium chloride: first choice
Potassium bicarbonate: for RTA
Potassium phosphate: for phos replacement

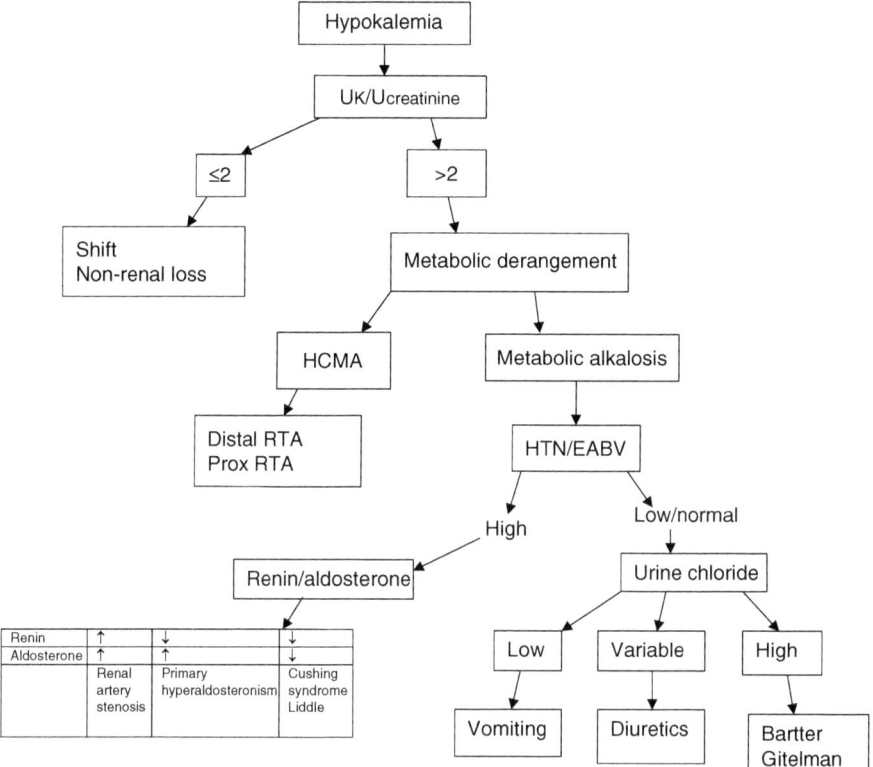

Fig. 4.1 Hypokalemia wkup. (Based on Kamel and Halperin [4]; Palmer and Clegg [2])

Hyperkalemia

For hyperkalemia, Table 4.4 for categories and Fig. 4.2 and Table 4.5 is the meds causing hyperkalemia due to RASS cascade interruption. Figure 4.3 for algorithm for hyperkalemia and K >6.5 mEq/L is a medical emergency to administer mediation quickly. Table 4.6 is for emergency medications and their onset of action.

Table 4.4   Causes of hyperkalemia

Etiology	Examples
Shift	Hemolysis
	Rhabdomyolysis
	TLS
	Lack of insulin
	Beta blockade
Renal failure	ESRD
	Mineralocorticoid deficiency
	Hyporenin hypoaldosteronism (Type 4 RTA)
Meds	ACEI/ARB
	K-sparing diuretic
	NSAID
	Heparin
	tacrolimus

Gennari [1]; Palmer and Clegg [2]

Fig. 4.2   Drugs causing hyperkalemia and mechanism

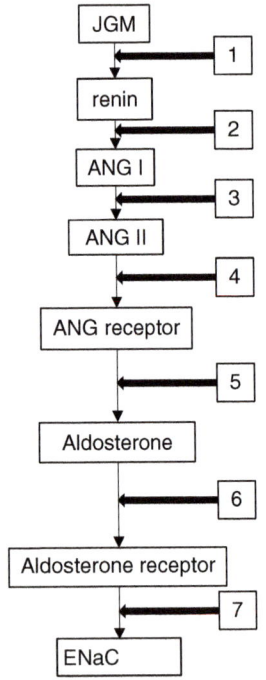

Table 4.5 RAAS casade interruption and medications

	Mechanism of action	Medications
1	Impaired release of renin	NSAID, CIN
2	Direct renin inhibitor	
3	ANG converting enzyme inhibitor	ACEi
4	ANG receptor blocker	ARB
5	Impaired aldosterone metabolism	Heparin, ketoconazole
6	ALD receptor blocker	MRA
7	ENaC blocker	Amiloride, triamterene, trimethoprim, pentamidine

Palmer and Clegg [2]

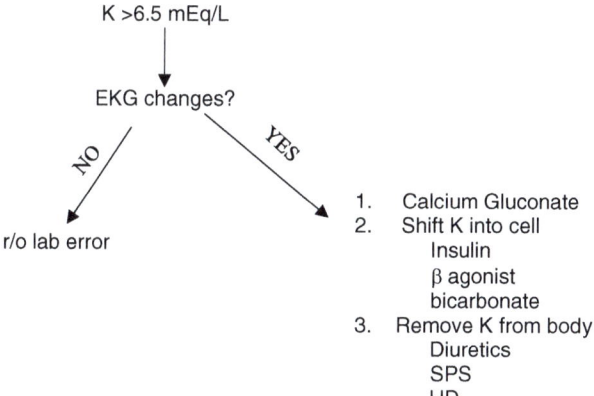

Fig. 4.3 Tx for hyperkalemia [5]

Table 4.6 Treatment modalities for hyperkalemia

Medication	Dose	Onset of action
Calcium gluconate	4.65 mEq IV	5–10 min
Insulin	10 U IV	15–20 min
Albuterol	20 mg nebulized	30–60 min
Sodium polystyrene sulfate (SPS)	15–30 g	Variable
Sodium bicarbonate	50 mmol/L	4–6 h

Shingarev and Allon [5]

References

1. ☺ ☺ ☺ Gennari F. Disorders of potassium homeostasis hypokalemia and hyperkalemia. Crit Care Clin. 2002;18:273–88.
2. ☺ ☺ ☺ Palmer B, Clegg D. Physiology and pathophysiology of potassium homeostasis. Adv Pshysiol Edu. 2016;40:480–90.
3. Faubel S, Topf J. The fluid, electrolyte & acid-base companion. San Diego: Alert and Oriented Publishing Co; 1999.
4. ☺ ☺ Kamel K, Halperin M. Use of urine electrolytes and urine osmolality in the clincial diagnosis of fluid, electrolyges, and acid-base disorders. Kidney Int Rep. 2021;6:1211–24.
5. ☺ Shingarev R, Allon M. A physiologic-based approach to the treatment of acute hyperkalemia. Am J Kidney Dis. 2010;56(3):578–84.

Minerals

5

Table 5.1 Overview

	Calcium		Phosphorus		Magnesium	
	↑	↓	↑	↓	↑	↓
3× Etiology						
1	↑ GI absorption TB/HIV/MAC	GI loss (vit D low)	↓ Renal excretion Low GFR Thyrotoxicosis Hypoparathyroidism	GI loss Etoh	CKD	GI loss PPI use Diarrhea
2	↑ Bone resorption ↑ PTH, malignancy	↓ Bone resorption (low PTH)	Phos load Endogenous TLS, rhabdomyolysis, hemolysis Exogenous Vit D intoxication	Renal loss PHPT Vit D def	Mg load Meds (Table 5.4) Laxatives antacids	Renal loss Meds Aminoglycosides Tacrolimus Hypercalcemia
3	↓ Renal excretion Li, HCTZ	Shift Acute pancreatitis TLS	Pseudo Paraproteinemia (multiple myeloma)	Shift Respiratory alkalosis Refeeding syndrome DKA	Salt water drowning	Shift Refeeding syndrome Hungry bone syndrome Hyperthyroidism
Symptom	"Stones, bones, moans, and groans" (Table 5.2)	Enhanced neuromuscular activation: Chvostek, Trousseau	Due to hypocalcemia	Myocardial dysfunction if sever	Neuromuscular + cardiac toxicity	Neuromuscular and cardiac
Dx	PTH, vit D (Fig. 5.1)	PTH, Mg, vit D, phos (Table 5.3)		PTH, vitD, calcium		(Figure 5.2 and Table 5.4)
Tx	Volume expansion Calcitonin bisphosphonate	"Rule of 10" 10% calcium gluconate 10 ml over 10 min	Sevelamer and other phos binder	Not clear if need tx unless on vent IV phos can cause hypocal	Calcium administration IV in hypotension and resp. depression furosemide	Oral mg chloride or mg lactate

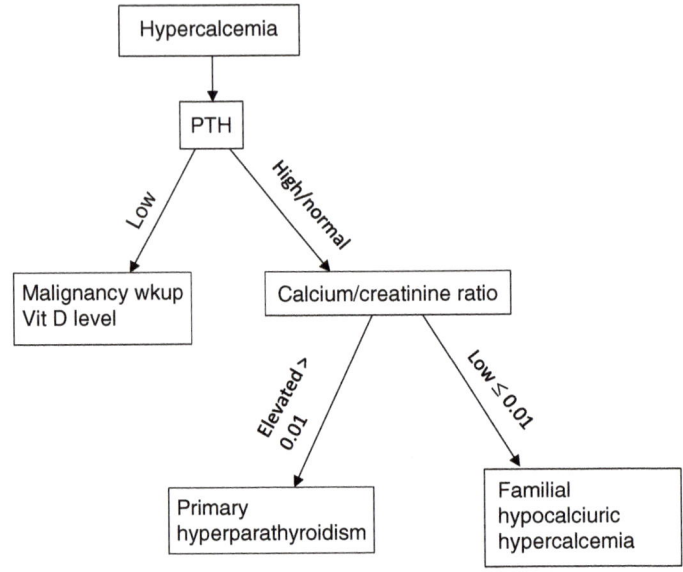

Fig. 5.1 Hypercalcemia. (Based on Carrol and Schade [1]; Michels and Kelly [2]; Minisola et al. [3])

Table 5.2 Stones, bones, moans, and groans

Renal "**stones**"	Nephrolithiasis
	Neph DI
Skeleton "**bones**"	Bone pain
	Arthritis
	Osteoporosis
GI "Abdominal **moans**"	N/V
	Abdominal pain
	Pancreatitis
	PUD
"Psychic **groans**"	Impaired concetration/memory
	Confusion, lethargy
	Muscle weakness
	Corneal calcification
CVD	HTN
	Vascular calcification

Carroll and Schade [1]

Table 5.3 Hypocalcemia

Steps		Decision	Condition
	Hypocalcemia		
1	Magnesium ⟶	If low ⟶	Treathypomagnesemia
2	Phosphorus ⟶	If low ⟶	Vit D deficiency
3	PTH ⟶	If low ⟶	Hypoparathyroidism
		If high ⟶	Pseudohypoparathyroidism CKD

Cooper and Gittoes [4]; Jain and Reilly [5]

- The most common cause of hypocalcemia is vitamin D def [4]
- Trousseau's sign is more specific than Chvostek's [4]

Hyperphosphatemia
- Most commonly results from CKD (>90% of cases) [5]

Hypophosphatemia
- Phos is low with calcium, then check vitamin D (Hypocalcemia workup above)

Hypermagnesemia
- CKD and exogenous source as above table

Hypomagnesemia

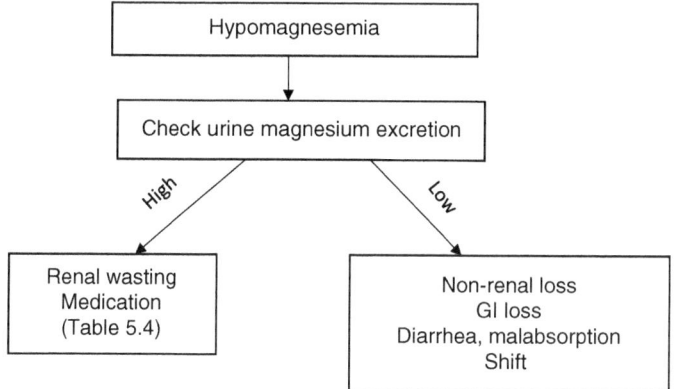

Fig. 5.2 Hypomagnesemia. (Based on Reilly [6]; Adomako and Yu [7])

Table 5.4 Meds related to hypomagnesemia

Diretics	Osmotic diuretics
	Loop
	HCTZ
Epidermal growth factor receptor modulators	Cetuximab
	Erlotinib
Antimicrobials	Aminoglycoside
	Amphotericin B
CIN	Cyclosporine
	FK506
others	Sirolimus
	Cisplatic
	Pentamidine
	Foscarnet
	PPI [8]

Dimke et al. [9]

References

1. ☺☺☺Carroll M, Schade D. A practical approach to hypercalcemia. Am Fam Physician. 2003;67:1959–66.
2. Michels T, Kelly K. Parathyroid disorders. Am Fam Physician. 2013;88(4):249–57.
3. ☺Minisola S, et al. The diagnosis and management of hypercalcemia. BMJ. 2015;350:h2723. https://doi.org/10.1136/bmj.h2723.
4. ☺☺☺Cooper M, Gittoes N. Diagnosis and management of hypocalcemia. BMJ. 2008;336:1298–302.
5. Jain N, Reilly R. Disorders of calcium homeostasis – hypo and hypercalcemia. In: Reilly R, Perazella M, editors. Nephrology in 30 days. McGraw Hill Medical; 2014. p. 133–48.
6. Reilly R. Disorders of magnesium homeostasis – hypo and hypermagnesemia. In: Reilly R, Perazella M, editors. Nephrology in 30 days. McGraw Hil Medical; 2014. p. 165–77.
7. ☺☺Adomako E, Yu A. Magnesium disorders: Core curriculum 2024. Am J Kidney Dis. 2024;83(6):803–15.
8. Danziger J, et al. Proton-pump inhibitor use is associated with low serum magnesium concentrations. Kidney Int. 2013;83:692–9.
9. ☺☺Dimke H, et al. Evaluation of hypomagnesemia: lessons from disorders of tubular transport. Am J Kidney Dis. 2013;62(2):377–83.

Fluid

6

Flowchart

```
                    ┌─────────────┐
                    │    Fluid    │
                    └──────┬──────┘
                           ▼
        ┌──────────────────────────────────────┐
        │ Fluid compartment in our body (Fig. 6.1) │
        └──────────────────┬───────────────────┘
                           ▼
        ┌──────────────────────────────────────┐
        │   Dehydration vs volume depletion    │
        └──────────────────┬───────────────────┘
                           ▼
        ┌──────────────────────────────────────┐
        │        Colloid vs crystalloid        │
        └──────────────────┬───────────────────┘
                           ▼
        ┌──────────────────────────────────────┐
        │        Fluid responsiveness          │
        └──────────────────┬───────────────────┘
                           ▼
        ┌──────────────────────────────────────┐
        │    Complication of fluid overload    │
        └──────────────────────────────────────┘
```

Fig. 6.1 Fluid compartment in our body

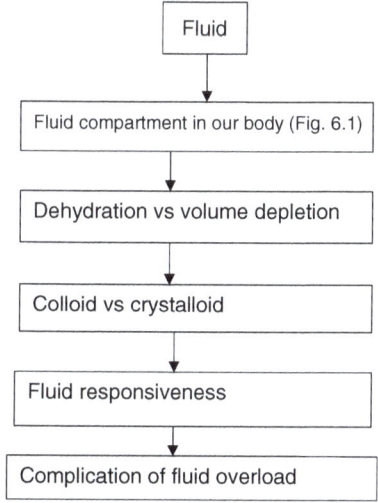

- 85% of blood in venous side, 15% on arterial side [1]

Hypovolemia has 2 forms:

1. Volume depletion
2. Dehydration

- Volume depletion (loss of sodium from extracellular space (Intravascular and interstitial fluid) ((Na loss)) (elevated serum urea nitrogen/creatinine ratio)
- Dehydration (loss of intracellular water that ultimately cause cellular desiccation and hypernatremia and hyperosmolality) ((Hypernatremia)) (elevated serum sodium level or osmolality level)

Endothelium (beyond Sterling Law)

Endothelial glycocalyx [2, 3]
- Crystalloid have not ability to restore the endothelial glycocalyx, but FFP may have restoring properties [3]
- Inflammation disrupts glycocalyx layer and promotes loss of plasma fluid to interstitial space [4] (Fig. 6.2)

Fig. 6.2 Endothelial glycocalyx layer

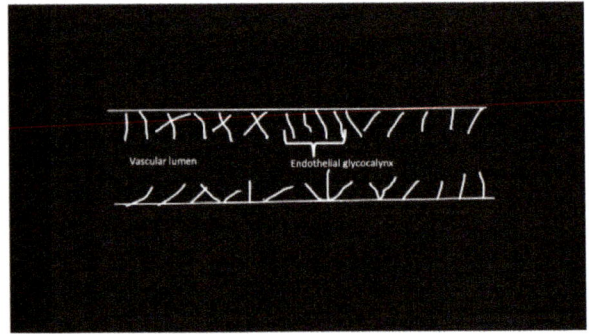

Colloid vs crystalloid
- Two occasions we prefer colloid for resuscitation

    1. Liver cirrhosis
    2. Early septic shock

- One condition we should avoid colloid
    1. TBI
- Approximately 60% of the infused fluid volume diffuses int the interstitial compartment within 20 min of administration [5]

Crystalloid composition [6]

Fluid	Sodium	Potassium	Chloride	Osmolarity
LR	130	4.0	109	273
0.9% NS	154	–	154	308

Fluid administration
- Isotonic fluid may result in hyponatremia in CNS injury who has cerebral salt wasting or has SIADH, those urine osmolality >500 mOsm/kg
- Only isotonic solution should be used for maintenance IV fluid considering high prevalence of elevated AVP level among hospitalized patients [7]

Default maintenance solution for adult is D5 NS at 100–120 ml/h

Or

Holliday-Segar formula

First 10 kg	100 ml/kg
Second 10 kg	50 ml/kg
The rest	25 ml/kg

Holliday and Segar [8]

Fluid responsiveness
- PLR [9]
- Responders >15% change in SV [10]
- Real time SV monitoring with PLR maneuver or fluid challenge is the only accurate method to evaluate fluid responsiveness [11, 12]

Fluid overload
- With systemic inflammation, the loss of fluid in intravascular space into interstitial space is not simply dictated by plasma oncotic pressure, but glycocalyx integrity.
- Pathologic sequalae of fluid overload in organs [4]
- Each 1% increase in % fluid overload at RRT initiation, risk of death will increase by 3% [13].
- Sodium rich and chloride rich solutions (ie NS) may trigger afferent arteriolar vasoconstriction via tubuloglomerular feedback.
- Effect of fluid overload in kidney [14]
- Fluid overload impairs anastomotic healing [15]
- Excessive fluid resuscitation increased the incidence of postoperative complications [16]
- For traumatic hemorrhagic shock, damage control resuscitation [17]

References

1. Schrier R. Decreased effective blood volume in edematous disorders: what does this mean? J Am Soc Nephrol. 2007;18:2028–31.
2. ☺☺☺Myburgh J, Mythen M. Resuscitation fluid. N Engl J Med. 2013;369:1243–51.
3. Milford E, Reade M. Resuscitation fluid choices to preserve the endothelial glycocalyx. Crit Care. 2019;23:77. https://doi.org/10.1186/s13054019-2369-x.
4. ☺☺O'Connor M, Prowle J. Fluid overload. Crit Care Clin. 2015;31:803–21.
5. Varrier M, Ostermann M. Fluid composition and clinical effects. Crit Care Clin. 2015;31:823–37.
6. Semier M, Kellum J. Balanced crystalloid solutions. Am J Respir Crit Care Med. 2019;199(8):952–60.
7. ☺☺Moritz M, Ayus J. Maintenance intravenous fluids in acutely ill patients. N Engl J Med. 2015;373:1350–60.
8. Holliday M, Segar W. The maintenance need for water in parenteral fluid therapy. Pediatrics. 1957;19:823–32.
9. Monnet X, Teboul J. Passive leg raisin: five rules, not a drop of fluid! Crtical Care. 2015. https://doi.org/10.1186/s13054-014-0708-5.
10. Preau S, et al. Passive leg raising is predictive of fluid responsiveness in spontaneously breathing patients with severe sepsis or acute pancreatitis. Crit Care Med. 2010;38:819–25.
11. ☺☺Bentzer P, et al. Will this hemodynamically unstable patient respond to a bolus of intravenous fluids? JAMA. 2016;316(12):1298–309.
12. ☺Marik P. Fluid responsiveness and the six guiding principles of fluid resuscitation. Crit Care Med. 2016;44(10):1920–2.
13. Rewa O, Bagshaw S. Principles of fluid management. Crit Care Clin. 2015;31:785–801.
14. ☺☺☺Glassford N, Bellomo R. Does fluid type and amount affect kidney function in critical illness? Crit Care Clin. 2018;34:279–98.
15. Lobo D. Flulid overload and surgical outcome. Ann Surg. 2009;249:186–8.
16. Futier E, et al. Conservative vs restrictive individualized goal-directed fluid replacement strategy in major abdominal surgery. A prospective randomized trial. Arch Surg. 2010;145:1193–200.
17. Chang R, Holcomb J. Optimal fluid therapy for traumatic hemorrhagic shock. Crit Care Clin. 2017;33:15–36.

Nutrition

7

Flowchart

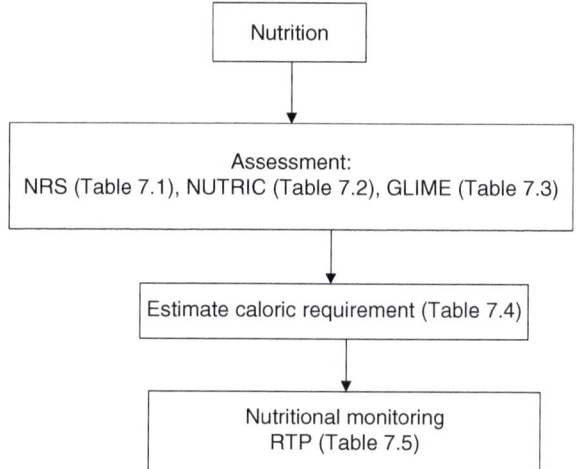

Fact:

- Hospitalized patients are at risk of malnutrition due to Disease-related malnutrition (DRM) [1]

Assessment tool [2]: NRS 2002, NUTRIC

- At risk: NRS ≥3, NUTRIC >4

© The Author(s), under exclusive license to Springer Nature Switzerland AG 2025
M. J. Morikawa, *The Inpatient Medicine Handbook*,
https://doi.org/10.1007/978-3-032-08398-2_7

Table 7.1 NRS (nutritional risk screening) [3]

• Based on 2 elements: nutritional status and disease severity		
• Score ≥3 (age-corrected): needs nutritional support		
Nutritional status	Disease severity	Score
Normal nutritional status	Normal nutritional requirements	0
Wt loss >5% in 3 months Foot intake <50–75% of normal requirements in proceeding week	Hip fracture Acute on chronic LC, COPD, DM, HD or oncology problems	1
Wt loss >5% in 2 months BMI 18.5–20.5 + impaired general condition Food intake 25–50% of normal requirement in proceeding week	Major abdominal surgery CVA Severe CAP, hematologic malignancy	2
Wt loss >5% in 1 months BMI <18.5 + general deconditioning Food intake 0–25% of normal requirements in proceeding week	Head injury BM transplant ICU (APACHE 10)	3

- Add (nutritional status score) + (disease severity score)
- If age ≥70, add 1 to total score to correct for frailty of elderly
- Score ≥3 start nutritional support

Table 7.2 NUTRIC score [4–6]

NUTRIC variable	Points
Age	
<50	0
50–<75	1
75≤	2
APACHE II score	
<15	0
15–<20	1
20≤	2
SOFA	
<6	0
6–<10	1
10≤	2
# of comorbidities	
0–1	0
2≤	1
Days from hospital to ICU admit	
<1	0
1≤	1
IL-6 (ng/mL)	
0–<400	0
400≤	1

- Total score 0–4: low risk
- 5–9: high risk needs aggressive nutritional support

Table 7.3 GLIM criteria for diagnosis of malnutrition [7, 8]

Malnutrition = One phenotypic criterion + one etiologic criterion

Phenotype criteria

Weight loss (%)	Low BMI	Reduced muscle mass
>5% within past 6 months or > 10% beyond 6 months	<20 if <70 years <22 if >70 years Asia: <18.5 if <70 years <20 if >70 years	Reduced by validated body composition measuring techniques

Etiologic criteria

Reduced food intake or assimilation	Inflammation
≤50% of energy requirement >1 week Any reduction >2 weeks Any chronic GI condition that adversely impacts food assimilation or absorption	Acute disease/injury Chronic illnesses

- Severity grading is based on phenotypic criterion

	Weight loss (%)	Low BMI	Reduced muscle mass
Stage 1: moderate	5–10% within the past 6 months or 10–20% beyond 6 months	<20 if <70 years <22 if ≥70 years	Mild to moderate deficit
Stage 2: severe	>10% within the past 6 months or >20% beyond 6 months	<18.5 if <70 years <20 if ≥70 years	Severe deficit

Table 7.4 Calorie requirement [9]

Total energy expenditure (TEE) = 27 kcal × body weight (kg)/day
Underweight patient = 30 × BW (kg)/day
Protein 1 g/kg/day

There are several ways to estimate resting metabolic rate (RMR):

- Mifflin-St Jeor equation [10] is the most accurate [11]
- Most hospitalized patients required 100–120% of BEE [12]

- Children >5 years [13]

1500 Kcal for the first 20 kg + 25 kcal/additional kg/day

Table 7.5 Nutritional monitoring: Rapid Turnover Protein (RTP)

Protein	Half life
Transferrin (TIBC × 0.8–43)	9 days
Prealbumin	2–4 days
Retinol-binding protein	12 hours

References

1. Bounoure L, et al. Detection and treatment of medical inpatients with or at-risk of malnutrition: suggested procedures based on validated guidelines. Nutrition. 2016;32:790–8.
2. ☺ ☺ ☺Schuetz P, et al. Management of disease-related malnutrition for patients being trated in hospital. Lancet. 2021;398:1927–38.
3. Kondrup J, et al. Nutritional risk screening (NRS 2002): a new method based on an analysis of controlled clinical trials. Clin Nutr. 2003;22(3):321–36.
4. Heyland D, et al. Identifying critcally ill patients who benefit the most from nturition therapy: the development and initial validation of a novel risk assessment tool. Crit Care. 2011;15:R268.
5. Rahman A, et al. Identifying critically-ill patients who will benefit most from nutritional therapy: further validation of the "modified NUTRIC" nutritional risk assessment tool. Clin Nutr. 2016;35:158–62.
6. Patel J, et al. Critical care nutrition. Where's the evidence? Crit Care Clin. 2017;33:397–412.
7. Cederholm T, et al. GLIM criteria for the diagnosis of malnutrition - a consensus report from the global clinical nutrition community. Clin Nutr. 2019;38:1–9.
8. Jensen G, et al. GLIM criteria for the diagnosis of malnutrition: a consensus report from the global clinical nutrition community. J Parenter Enteral Nutr. 2019;43(1):32–40.
9. Gomes F, et al. ESPEN guidelines on nutritional support for polymorbid internal medicine patients. Clin Nutr. 2018;37:336–53.
10. Mifflin M, et al. A new predictive equation for resting energy expenditure in healthy individuals. Am J Clin Nutr. 1990;51:241–7.
11. Frankenfield D, et al. Comparison of predictive equations for resting metabolic rate in healthy nonobese and obese adults: a systematic review. J Am Diet Assoc. 2005;105:775–89.
12. Miles J. Energy expenditure in hospitalized patients: implications for nutritional support. Mayo Clin Proc. 2006;81:809–16.
13. Kulick D, Deen D. Specialized nutrition support. Am Fam Physician. 2011;83(2):173–83.

Inpatient Glycemic Control

8

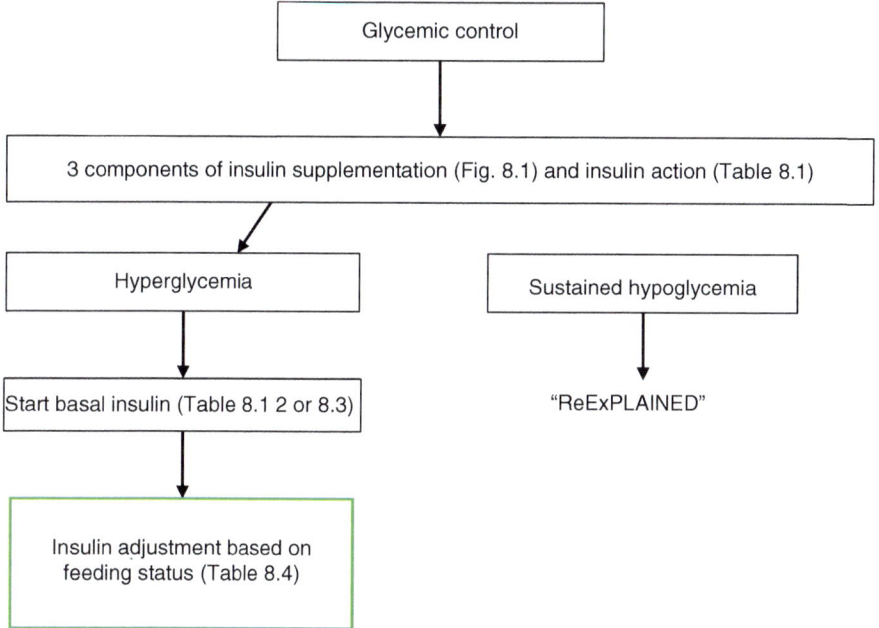

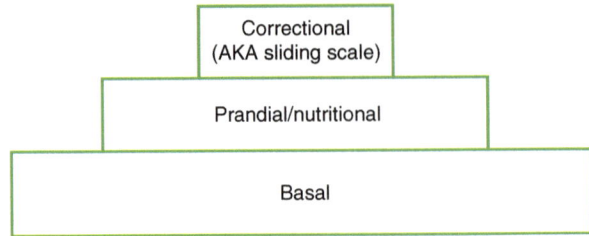

Fig. 8.1 Insulin supplementation is based on 3 components [1]

What is the 2 major downside of SSI coverage [2]?

1. Retroactive (causing roller coaster effect)
2. No survival benefit proven

Table 8.1 Duration of action of insulin [3]

	Onset	Peak	Duration of action
Basal			
NPH	1–3 h	6–8 h	12–16 h
Glargine	1–3 h	No peak	Up to 24 h
Detemir	1–3 h	No peak	Up to 24 h
Prandial			
Regular	15–60 min	2–4 h	6–8 h
Lispro	10–15 min	1 h	3–4 h
Aspart	10–15 min	1 h	3–4 h

$$\boxed{\text{Glycemic control goal} : 140 - 180\,\text{mg} / \text{dL}\,[3]}$$

Approach:

1. Estimate total daily dose (0.3–0.6 U/kg/day) [3]

Or

Table 8.2 Estimating total daily dose of insulin for insulin naïve hospitalized patients

Body habitus	Estimated units/kg
Normal weight	0.4
Stage IV CKD not HD	0.25
Underweight, old age or HD	0.3
Overweight	0.5
Obese, IR, or on steroid	≥0.6

Based on Kodner et al. [6]

2. 50% as basal and the other 50% in 3 split doses at meal time
3. Or

Table 8.3 "Miami 4/12" [4, 5]

| Basal insulin | Bodyweight (kg) ÷ 4 |
| Prandial insulin | Bodyweight (kg) ÷ 12 |

Table 8.4 Insulin adjustment depending on meals in inpatient [6]

Diet	Basal insulin (% of total daily insulin)	Nutritional insulin (% of total daily insulin)
Eating meals	50%	50%
NPO or clear liquid only	25%	–
Tube feeding (bolus or continuous)	40%	60%

Hypoglycemia

- Defined as BS <70 mg/dL [3]
- Sustained hypoglycemia, the following possibilities

"ReExPLAIND"

Re	Renal failure
Ex	Exogenous insulin
P	Pituitary problem
L	Liver failure
A	Adrenal failure
I	Infection is way more common than Insulinoma
N	Neoplasm such pancreatic cancer
D	Drugs: sulfonylurea, newer quinolone Abx are dysglycemic

References

1. Asudani D, Calles-Escandon J. Inpatient hyperglycemia: slide through the scale but cover the bases first. J Hosp Med. 2007;2(Suppl 1):23–32.
2. ☺ ☺ ☺Clement S, et al. Management of diabetes and hyperglycemia in hospitals. Diabetes Care. 2004;27:553–91.
3. ☺ ☺Horton W, Subauste J. Top 10 facts to know about inpatient glycemic control. Am J Med. 2016;129:139–42.
4. ☺ ☺Meneghini L. Intensifying insulin therapy: what options are available to patients with type 2 diabetes? Am J Med. 2013;126:S28–37.
5. Meneghini L. Perioperative management of diabetes: translating evidence into practice. Cleve Clin J Med. 2009;76(Suppl 4):S53–9.
6. Kodner C, et al. Glucose management in hospitalized patients. Am Fam Physician. 2017;96(10):648–54.

EKG/Cardiac Pacing

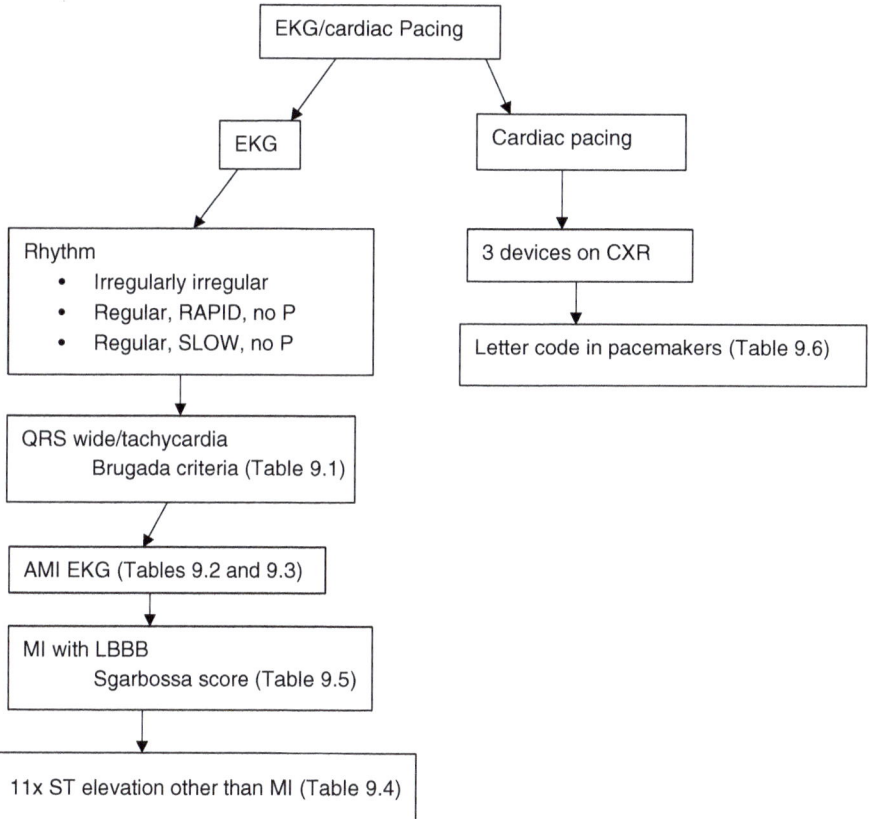

M. J. Morikawa, *The Inpatient Medicine Handbook*,
https://doi.org/10.1007/978-3-032-08398-2_9

Rhythm

1. If it's irregularly irregular, Atrial fibrillation
2. Rapid and regular, no P wave,

   1. SVT
   2. Sinus tach
   3. Atrial flutter

3. Slow and regular, no P wave,

   1. Junctional rhythm
   2. Digoxin toxicity
   3. Hyperkalemia

- Narrow QRS complex (<120 ms) with HR >100 is classified on the basis of RP interval. The RP internal represents the time from ventricular activation to atrial activation.
- Long RP tachycardias are (sinus tachycardia, focal atrial tachycardia) are separated from SVTs that have a short RP interval (AVNRT, orthodromic reciprocating tachycardia (ORT)) [1]

Wide QRS complex tachycardia

- Brugada criteria to differentiate SVT with aberrancy and VT [2, 3]

  Ask following questions in this order, if any yes, then VT, if all no, SVT with aberrancy.

Table 9.1 Brugada Criteria

1. RS complex absent from all precordial leads
2. RS complex present and R to S interval > 100 msec in 1 precordial lead
3. AV dissociation present
4. Morphologic criteria for VT present in precordial leads V1 to V2 and V6

AMI EKG [4]

Table 9.2 Inferior MI (RCA vs LCx)

RCA	ST elevation III > II + ST depression in I, aVL or both
RCA + RV infarction	Above + ST elevation in V1
LCx	ST elevation I, aVL, V5 and V6 + ST depression V1, V2, V3

Table 9.3 Anterior MI (L anterior descending A) = ST elevation V1, V2, V3 WITH

STelevation V1 > 2.5 mm or RBBB	Prox. L Ant Descending A
ST depression >1 mm in II, III, aVF	Prox. L ant descending A
ST depression ≤1 mm or ST elevation in II, III, aVF	Distal. Ant descending A

ST Changes

Table 9.4 10 causes of ST elevation other than MI [5]

1. male pattern
2. early repolarization
3. LBBB
4. pericarditis
5. Hyperkalemia
6. Brugada syndrome
7. PE
8. cardioversion
9. Prinzmetal's angina
10. V-paced
11. Takotsubo syndrome [6]

EKG Criteria for MI with LBBB [7, 8]

- Sgarbossa EKG score ≥ 3 is useful for diagnosing MI in LBBB

Table 9.5 Sgarbossa Score

EKG findings	Score
ST-segment elevation ≥ 1 mm and concordant with QRS complex	5
ST-segment depression ≥ 1 mm in lead V1, V2, or V3	3
ST-segment elevation ≥ 5 mm and discordant with QRS complex	2

Cardiac Pacing

You should be able to tell 3 different cardiac devices on CXR and their indications:

1. Cardiac pacer (Mostly **Dual-chamber** pacer)
2. ICD
3. Cardiac resynchronization therapy (CRT) (**Bi-ventricular** pacer)

Table 9.6 5-letter code in pacemakers [9]

- 1st letter: chamber that is paced (Atrium, ventricle, dual)
- 2nd letter: chamber sensed (Atrium, ventricle, dual)
- 3rd letter: the response to sensing (inhibit, trigger, dual)
- 4th letter: the presence or absence of rate modulation
- 5th letter: multisite pacing

ICD Shock

- Common causes of inappropriate shock are Af, SVT and sinus tachycardia. [10]
- Multiple shocks need emergency evaluation.

References

1. ☺ ☺ DeSimone C, et al. Supraventricular arrhythmias: clinical framework and common scenarios for the internist. Mayo Clin Proc. 2018;93(12):1825–41.
2. ☺ Brugada P, et al. A new approach to the differential diagnosis of a regular tachycardia with a wide QRS complex. Circulation. 1991;83:1649–59.
3. Helton M. Diagnosis and management of common types of supraventricular tachycardia. AFP. 2015;92(9):793–800.
4. ☺ ☺ Zimetbaum P, Josephson M. Use of the electrocardiogram in acute myocardial infarction. N Engl J Med. 2003;348:933–40.
5. ☺ ☺ ☺ Wang K, et al. ST-segment elevation in conditions other than acute myocardial infarction. N Engl J Med. 2003;349:2128–35.
6. Prasad A. Apical ballooning syndrome. An important differential diagnosis of acute myocardial infarction. Circulation. 2007;115:e56–9.
7. Sgarbossa E, et al. Electrocardiographic diagnosis of evolving acute myocardial infarction in the presence of left bundle-branch block. N Engl J Med. 1996;334:481–7.
8. Tobas J, et al. Electrocardiographic criteria for detecting acute myocardial infarction in patients with left bundle branch block: a meta-analysis. Ann Emerg Med. 2008;52:329–36.
9. ☺ ☺ Kaszala K, et al. Contemporary pacemakers: what the primary care physician needs to know. Mayo Clin Proc. 2008;83:1170–86.
10. Gehi A, et al. Evaluation and management of patients after implantable cardioverter-defibrillator shock. JAMA. 2006;296:2839–47.

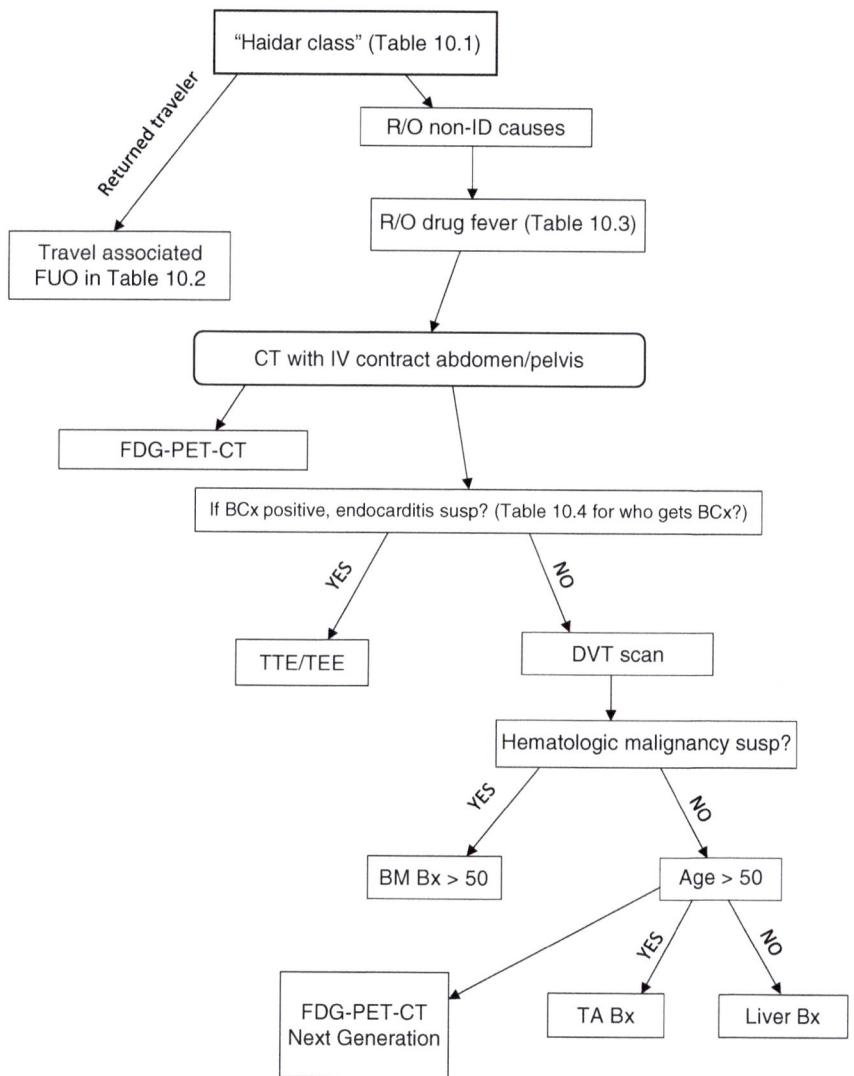

(Based on Haidar [1]; Mourad [2]; Varghese [3])

- Very high fever above 39.5 is not often caused by non-ID causes

Table 10.1 FUO "Haider class"

Categories	Examples
Classic	Infection (still most common up to 40%)
	Inflammation (up to 32%)
	Malignancy (up to 25%)
Nosocomial	CDI
Immunodeficiency-related	HIV
	Organ transplant recipient
	Hematologic cancer pt.
	On immunosuppressive therapies
Travel associated	Table 10.2 for DDx

Haidar [1]

Table 10.2 Travel associated FUO etiologies

First r/o malaria, then				
Viral		Bacterial		Parasitic
Arbovirus	Influenza	Bacteremia	Zoonotic	Hepatic
Dengue		Enteric	Spirochetal (leptospirosis,	amebiases
Chikungunya		fever	relapsing fever)	Schistosomiasis
Zika			Rickettsia	trypanosomiasis
Japanese			(typhus)	
encephalitis				

Bhargava (2018 fig. 1)

Table 10.3 Drugs-related FUO based on time of onset

types	Onset of fever	comments
Malignant hyperthermia	0.5–2.0 h	Depolarizing muscle relaxant and inhalation anesthetics
Mitochondrial uncoupling of oxidative phosphorylation	0.5–3.0 h	Pesticides and toxins
Infusion related reaction	0.5–3.0 h	Vancomycine, monoclonal abs
Anticholinergic fever	About 2 h	Anticonvulants; antiemetics, muscle relant, tricyclic antidepressant
Chemotherapy-related raction	3–19 h	Chemotherapeutic agents,
Serotonin syndrome (SS)	6 h— several days	SSRI, SNRI, tricyclic antidepressant, MAOI, serotonin receptor agonist
Hypersensitivity reaction	7–10 days	Antimicrobial agents, methyldopa, quinidine, allopurinol, anticonvulsant
Neuroleptic malignant syndrome (NMS)	1–2 weeks	Antipsycotic agents: haloperidol, quetiapine, olanzapine, reisperidone, antiemetics: metoclopramide, procholoperazine, abrupst withdrawal of dopamine agonists
DRESS	2–6 weeks	Sulfonamide, carbamazepine, allopurinol, lamotrigine, phenytoin
Adrenergic fever	Variable	Sympathomimetic agents and MAOI, cocaine, MDMA

(Modified from Haidar [1])

Table 10.4 Who needs blood cultures?

Severe sepsis/septic shock	Infective endocarditis/ endovascular infection is suspected	High Pretest prob. for bacteremia	Confirmation of clearance of bacteremia
		• CRBSI • discitis/native vertebrae osteomyelitis • epidural abscess • meningitis • nontraumatic septic arthritis • Ventriculoatrial shunt infection	• S. aureus, S. lugdunensis • bacteremia in endovascular infection • CRBSI before catheter replacement

Other Potential Indications

Intermediate pretest probabily patients with concerns for endovascular infection, or Bcx results impact mgmt.
- Actue pyelonephritis
- cholangitis
- Prostetic vertebral osteomyelitis
- severe CAP

Follow up BCx may need

- single + BCx with skin flora in symptomatic pts. with prostehsis or IV catheter
- concern for presisstent bacterial without source control

Fabre [4]

- Follow up Bcx added little value in the mgmt of GNB bacteremia [5]

References

1. ☺☺☺Haidar G, Singh N. Fever of unknown origin. N Engl J Med. 2022;386:463–77.
2. ☺☺☺Mourad O, et al. A comprehensive evidence-based approach to fever of unknown origin. Arch Intern Med. 2003;163:545–51.
3. Varghese G, et al. Investigating and managing pyrexia of unknown origin in adults. BMJ. 2010;341:878–81.
4. ☺☺Fabre V, et al. Does this patient need blood cultures? A scoping review of indications for blood cultures in adult nonneutropenic inpatients. Clin Inf Dis. 2020;71(5):1339–47.
5. ☺Canzoneri C, et al. Follow-up blood cultures in gram-negative bacteremia: are they needed? Clin Infect Dis. 2017;65(11):1776–9.

SEPSIS

11

SEPSIS-3 (2016)

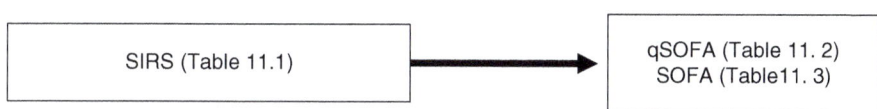

Fig. 11.1 Change in concept of sepsis: SIRS to SOFA [1]

Table 11.1 SIRS

SIRS (Systemic Inflammatory Response Syndrome)
Two or more of:
Temperature > 38 °C or < 36 °C
HR > 90 /min
RR > 20/min or PaCO2 < 32 mmHg
WBC >12,000/mm³ or < 4000/mm³ or > 10% immature bands

Table 11.2 qSOFA

qSOFA (quick SOFA) criteria
Altered mentation
RR ≥ 22 /min
SBP ≤ 100 mmHg

Table 11.3 SOFA; Sequential Organ Failure Assessment (SOFA) variables and score

	Score				
Variables	0	1	2	3	4
CNS GCS	15	13–14	10–12	6–9	6>
Resp RI (PaO2/FIO2 mmHg)	≥400	<400	<300	<200 or vent	<100 or vent
CVD MAP(mmHg) or pressor	≥70	<70	DOA < 5 or DOB any dose	DOA 5.1–15 or Epi ≤ 0.1 or Norepi≤0.1	DOA > 15 or Epi > 0.1 or Norepi>0.1
Liver Bilirubin (mg/dL)	<1.2	1.2–1.9	2.0–5.9	6.0–11.9	≥12.0
Renal Creatinine (mg/dL)or UO (ml/day)	<1.2	1.2–1.9	2.0–3.4	3.5–4.9 <500	≥5.0 <200
Coag Platelet (x103 µL)	≥150	<150	<100	<50	<20

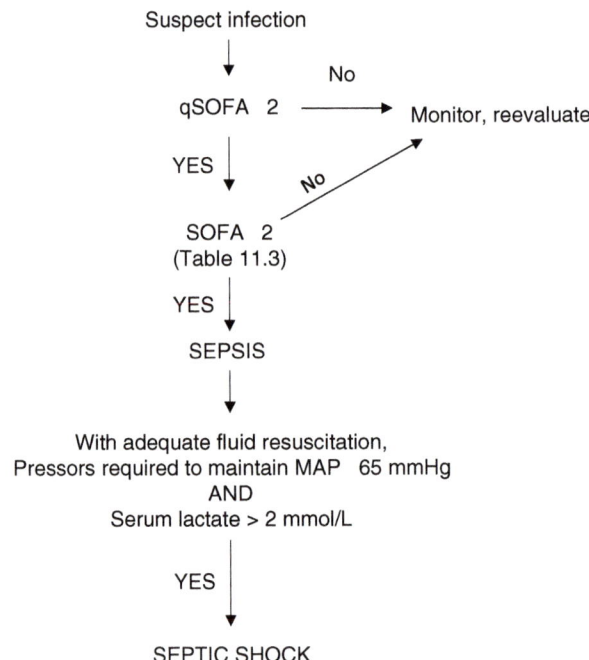

Fig. 11.2 Diagnostic procedure for sepsis, septic shock

Resuscitation: [2]

$$LR >>>> NS$$

Fluid responsiveness:

- Cap refill, Urine output
- Measure stroke volume with augmenting preload by passive leg raising (PLR), not IVC size

Enhancing recovery from sepsis [3]

- Delirium monitoring
- Pain assessment
- Early ambulation

Or

- Sleep, poop, appetite (SPA therapy)

References

1. ☺ ☺ ☺ Singer M, et al. The third international Concensus definitions for sepsis and septic shock (Sepsis-3). JAMA. 2016;315(8):801–10.
2. ☺ ☺ ☺ Ladzinski A, et al. Rational fluid resuscitation in sepsis for the hospitalist: a narrative review. Mayo Clin Proc. 2021;96(9):2464–73.
3. Prescott H, Angus D. Enhancing recovery from sepsis. A review. JAMA. 2018;319(1):62–75.

Acute Mental Status Change

12

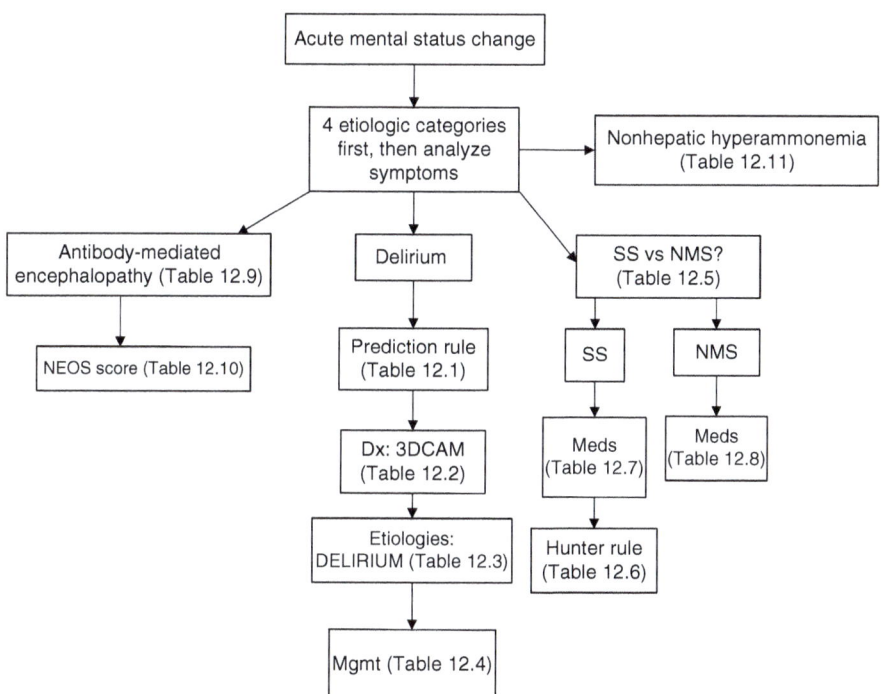

General

4 most common etiologies based on frequencies in the hospital [1]

1. Infection
2. Metabolic
3. Medication
4. Neurological

Delirium

Delirium clinical features [2, 3]

1. Fluctuating mental status
2. inattention
3. disorganized thinking
4. altered level of consciousness

Table 12.1 Delirium prediction score

Risk factors	Points
Vision impairment	1
Cognitive impairment	1
Severe illness (APACHE>16)	1
Elevated BUN/creatinine ratio (>18)	1

score	Risk
0	9%
1–2	23%
3–4	83%

Inouye et al. [4]; Miller [5]

Table 12.2 Delirium diagnostic tool: 3D- CAM

	Feature 1	Feature 2	Feature 3	Feature 4
Type of assessment	ΔMS with fluctuating course	Inattention	Disorganized thinking	Altered level of consciousness
Patient response	Being confused? Not in the hospital? Seeing things that are not really there?	Digit span 3 or 4 backward Days of the week backward Months of the year backward	The current year? The day of the week? The type of place?	None
Interviewer observation	Fluctuation in attention Fluctuation in speech or thinking	Trouble keeping track of the interview Easily distractable		Sleepy? Stuporous or comatose? Hypervigilant?

Delirium = feature 1 + feature 2 + either feature 3 or 4 (if feature 1 is uncertain, ask family or friend)
Marcantonio [6]; Wong et al. [7]

Table 12.3 Etiologies: "DELIRIUM"

D	Drugs interaction
E	Electrolytes disorder
L	Lack of drugs (inadequate pain control or withdrawal from alcohol or other meds
I	Infection
R	Reduced sensory input, poor vision, hearing
	Respiratory failure
I	Intracranial disorders (CVA, infection)
U	Urinary retention, fecal impaction
M	Myocardial and pulmonary diseases metabolic disorder (malnutrition, vit B12 def)

Marcantonio [6]; Nguyen et al. [8]

Table 12.4 Pharmacologic mgmt [9]

Mgmt of severe agitation	dose
Seroquel	12.5–25 mg PO BID
Olanzapine	2.5–5 mg PO BID
Risperidone	0.5–1 mg PO BID
Haloperidol	0.25–0.5 mg PO/IV
Mgmt of sleep wake cycle	
Melatonin	3–5 mg PO QHS
Ramelteon	8 mg PO QHS

In mgmt of behavioral and psychological symptoms of dementia (BPSD),

- For BPSD, citalopram and sertraline is well tolerated
- NMDA antagonist (Memantine) is useful to treat hallucinations, agitation and aggression [8]

Table 12.5 SS/NMS/anticholinergic syndrome

	Serotonin syndrome	Neuroleptic malignant syndrome (NMS)	Anticholinergic toxicity
Reflex	Hyper	Hypo	Normal
Pupil	Dilated (mydriasis)	normal	Dilated
Mental status	Agitation		Agitation
Skin	diaphoresis		Dry
Muscle	Increased tone: clonus Greater in lower extremities	RIGIDITY (Lead-pipe rigidity)	Urinary retention
Bowel sound	Hyperactive, diarrhea	Normal, decreased	Absent
Diagnostic tool	Hunter's criteria [10, 11]	Levenson's criteria	
	Clonus, ocular clonus Hyperreflexia Agitation, diaphoresis	Fever, rigidity, CK elevation	

Based on Boyer and Shannon [12]; Bienvenu et al. [13]; Bhanushali and Tuite [14]

Table 12.6 Hunter's decision rules for SS

Ask following questions in this order, if any of the answers yes, then SS, if no yes, then no SS
1. Spontaneous clonus
2. Inducible clonus + agitation or diaphoresis
3. Ocular clonus + agitation or diaphoresis
4. Tremor + hyperreflexia
5. Hypertonia+temp>38 °C + ocular or inducible clonus

Table 12.7 Meds contribute to SS [10]

Categories	Meds
Antidepressants/mood stabilizers	Buspirone
	MAO inhibitors
	Lithium
	SSRI
	SNRI
	Tricyclic antidepressant
	Serotonin 2A receptor blockers
antiemetics	Metoclopramide
	Ondansetron
Antimigraine meds	Carbamazepine
	Triptans
	Valproic acid
	Ergot
Analgesics	Cyclobenzaprine
	Fentanyl
	Tramadol
Amphethamine and derivatives	Methamphetamine
	Dextroamphetamine
	Ecstasy
others	Cocaine
	Dextromethorphan
	linezolid

Table 12.8 Medications associated with NMS

- Reduced dopamine neurotransmission centrally either by discontinuation or initiation of medications
- Most cases of NMS are with haloperidol and depot fluphenazine.

Withdrawal from	Induction of
Levodopa	Neuroleptics (haloperidol, fluphenazine, droperidol)
Dopamine agonists	Atypical antipsychotics (clozapine, olanzapine, risperidone, quetiapine)
Amantadine	Dopamine blockers (metoclopramide, prochlorperazine, promethazine)
	Tricyclic overdose, cocaine, amphetamine

Bienvenu et al. [13]; Bhanushali and Tuite [14]

Antibody-Mediated Encephalitis [15]

- Two potential triggers of autoimmune encephalitis are tumors and viral encephalitis [15]

Table 12.9 Main types of autoimmune encephalitis

• Treatment: steroid, IgIV, immunotherapy					
	Limbic	Anti-NMDAR	ADEM	Anti-GFAP	Anti-GABAAR
Epi/history	Adults subacute	Children/young adults Female Subacute or acute	Children/young adults Acute	Children/young adults Acute	Children/young adults Subacute or acute
Etiology	Tumor (50–95%)	Tumor HSV	Systemic infection vaccination	unknown	unknown
Signs	Memory deficit Seizures Psychiatric symptoms	Behavioral change Psychosis Movement disorders Autonomic dysfunction	Encephalopathy Fever Myelopathy Optic neuritis	Encephalopathy Fever Myelopathy Optic neuritis	Seizures Refractory status epilepticus
Abx	Anti-LGI1, GABAB-R or AMPA-R in CSF or serum	Anti-NMDAR in CSF	Anti-MOG in serum	Anti-GFAP in CSF	Anti-GAAAR in CSF or serum

Sonneville et al. [16]

Table 12.10 NEOS Score: Anti-NMDA receptor encephalitis 1-year functional status prediction

Variables and score points	
Variable	points
ICU admission required	1
No clinical improvement after 4 wk. of tx	1
No treatment <4 wk. of symptom onset	1
Abnormal MRI	1
CSF WBC > 20 cells/µL	1

NOES score	Good functional status at 1-year (mRS < 3) (%)
0–1	95<
2	90
3	70
4–5	30

Balu et al. [17]

Table 12.11 NONHEPATIC HYPERAMMONEMIA

Etiologies	Examples
Medications	Valproic acid
	Chemotherapy
Infection	Urease-producing bacteria
Recent surgery	Lung transplant
	Bariatric surgery
	Ureterosigmoidoscopy
Hyperalimentation	
Errors of metabolism	Urea cycle enzyme deficiency
	]fatty acid oxidation defects
	Amino acid transport defect

LaBuzetta et al. [18]

References

1. Jha A, Shojania K. Forgotten but not gone. N Engl J Med. 2004;350:2399–404.
2. ☺ ☺ ☺ Young J, Inouye S. Delirium in older people. BMJ. 2007;334:842–6.
3. Kalish V, et al. Delirium in older persons: evaluation and management. AFP. 2014;90(3):150–8.
4. Inouye S, et al. A predictive model for delirium in hospitalized elderly medical patients based on admission characteristics. Ann Intern Med. 1993;119:474–81.
5. Miller M. Evaluation and management of delirium in hopsitalized older patients. AFP. 2008;78:1265–70.
6. Marcantonio E. Delirium in hospitalized older adults. N Engl J Med. 2017;377:1456–66.
7. Wong C, et al. Does this patient have delirium? Value of bedside instruments. JAMA. 2010;304(7):779–86.
8. Nguyen J, et al. Ward based management of behavioural and spychological symptoms of dementia. BMJ. 2021;374:n1779. https://doi.org/10.1136/bmj.n1779.
9. Oh E, et al. Delirium in older persons. Advances in diagnosis and treatment. JAMA. 2017;318(12):1161–74.
10. Ables A, Nagubilli R. Prevention, diagnosis, and management of serotonin syndrome. AFP. 2010;81(9):1139–42.
11. Dunkley E, et al. The hunter serotonix toxicity criteria: simple and accurate diagnostic decision rules for serotonin toxicity. Q J Med. 2003;96(9):635–42.
12. Boyer E, Shannon M. The serotonin syndrome. N Engl J Med. 2005;352:1112–20.
13. Bienvenu O, et al. Treatment of four psychiatric emergencies in the intensive care unit. Crit Care Med. 2012;40:2662–70.
14. Bhanushali M, Tuite P. The evaluation and management of patients with neuroleptic malignant syndrome. Neurol Clin North Am. 2004;22:389–411.
15. Dalmau J, Graus F. Antibody-mediated encephalitis. N Engl J Med. 2018;378:840–51.
16. ☺ ☺ Sonneville R, et al. Understanding auto-immune encephalitis in the ICU. Intensive Care Med. 2019;45:1795–8.
17. Balu RM, McCracken L, et al. A score that predicts 1-year functional status in patients with anti-NMDA receptor encephalitis. Neurology. 2019;92:e244–52.
18. LaBuzetta J, et al. Adult nonhepatic hyperammonemia: a case report and diffential diagnosis. Am J Med. 2010;123:885–91.

Acute Kidney Injury (AKI)

13

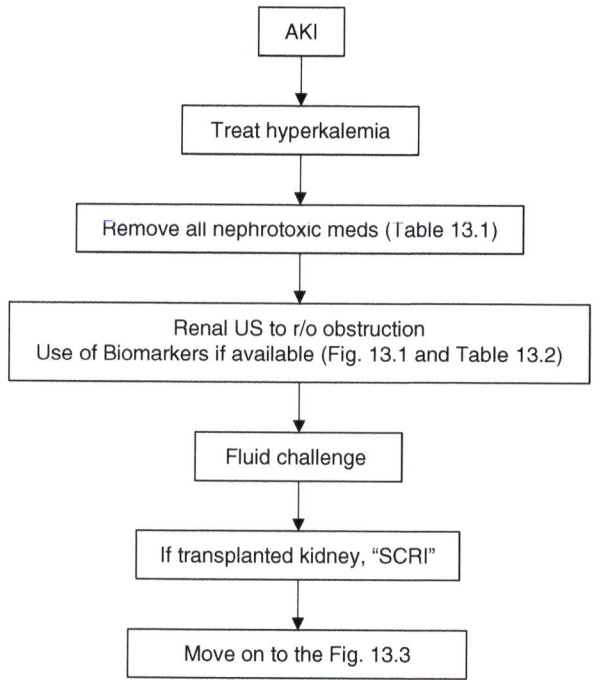

Fig. 13.1 AKI: Do this now!

Table 13.1 Medications affecting AKI

Aminoglycosides
NSAIDs
ACEI/ARB
Amphotericin
Cisplatin
Foscarnet
Iodinated contrast
Pentamidine
Tenofovir
Zolendronic acid

(Mercado et al. [1]; Moore et al. [2]; Pannu and Nadim [3])

M. J. Morikawa, *The Inpatient Medicine Handbook*,
https://doi.org/10.1007/978-3-032-08398-2_13

AKI in Transplant kidney **"Serum Creatinine IncRease"**
S: structural: anastomosis failure (hydronephrosis, renal doppler)
C: calcineurin inhibitor
I: infection including CMV, BK virus
R: Rejection

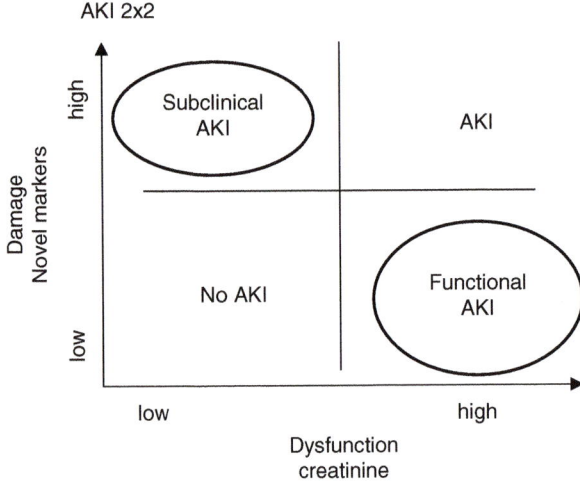

Fig. 13.2 Use of novel biomarkers
Based on Kulvichit et al. [4]

Table 13.2 AKI Biomarkers

Function	Biomarkers
Glomerular function	Creatinine
	Cystatin C
Inflammation	IL-18
	Proenkephalin
Tubular damage	NGAL
	KIM-1
	L-FABP

Based on Ostermann and Joannidis [5]; Belcher et al. [6]; Ronco et al. [7]

GFR estimation by creatinine clearance [8, 9]

Cockcroft-Gault Equation

$$Ccr\left(mL/min\right) = \left(140 - age\right) \times wt\left(kg\right) / \left(72 \times Scr\right) \times \left(0.85\,if\,female\right)$$

Ccr: creatinine clearance, Scr: serum creatinine (mg/dL)

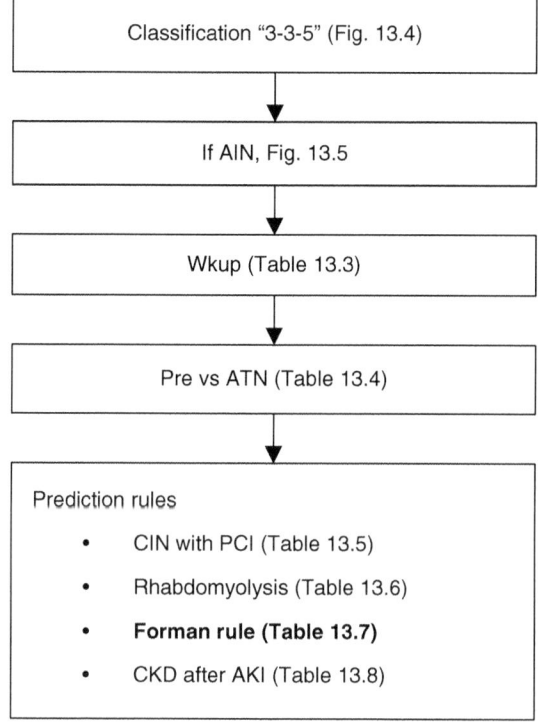

Fig. 13.3 AKI workup flowcharT
Classification: (Sethi et al. [10]; Lameire et al. [11]; Osterman and Joannidis [5])

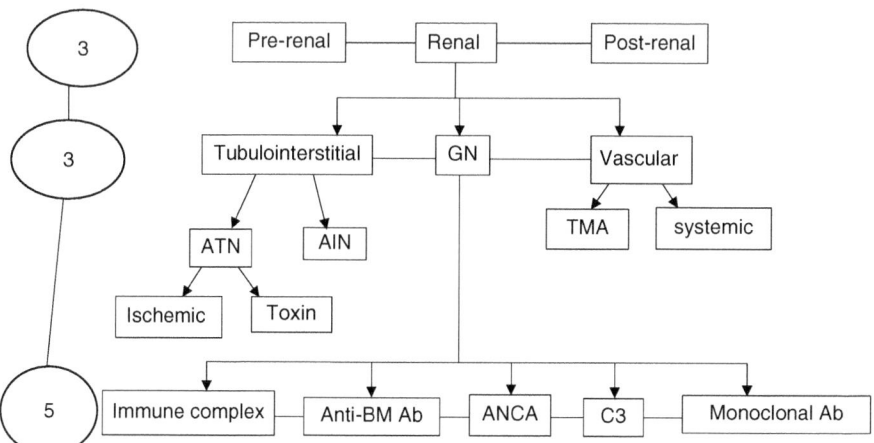

Fig. 13.4 "3-3-5" classification

Table 13.3 Workup

History	Nephrotoxic meds; malignancy
Clinical exam	Volume status; alveolar hemorrhage; abdominal symptoms; skin lesions e.g. purpura, petechiae
2D Echo	LV/RV/SHD
Renal US	Hydronephrosis/perfusion (contrast enhanced US) VExUS scan
Urinalysis	Proteinuria/hematuria/WBC/cast/Ucx
Blood work GN workup	Calcium; LFT;chem 7; platelet;DIC lab;hyperproteinemia; uric acid; CK
Urine	RBC cast, urinalysis, proteinuria quantification
Blood work	C3, C4, anti-dsDNA, ANCA, hepatitis panel, HIV, monoclonal protein, CRP, cryoglobulins, RA

Darmon et al. [12]

Table 13.4 prerenal vs ATN

	Prerenal	Renal ATN
BUN/Cr ratio	> 20	10–15
UA	Hyaline cast	Granular casts (muddy-Brown)
UNa	< 25 mEq/L	> 40 mEq/
FENa	< 1%	> 2%
UOsm	> 500 mOsm/kg	300–350 mOsm/kg
FEUrea	<35%	>50%

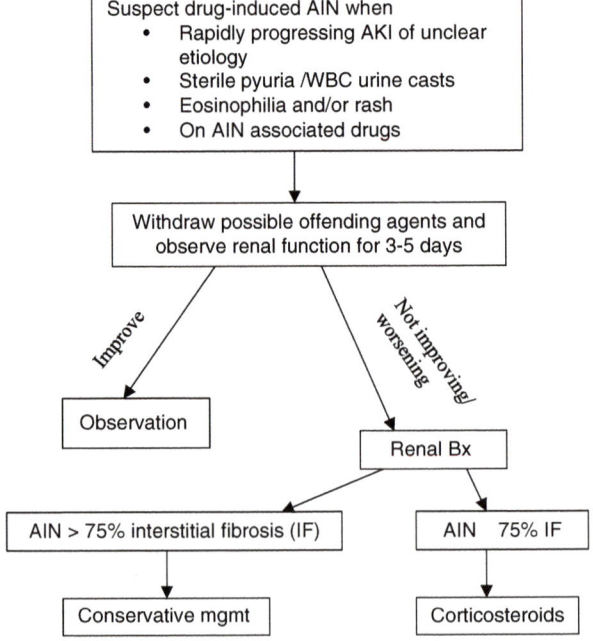

Fig. 13.5 Drug-induced AIN algorithm
(Based on Moledina and Perazella [13])

Prediction Rules

- CIN with PCI and prevention (Table 13.5)
- Rhabdomyolysis (Table 13.6)
- WRF with HF "Forman Rule" (Table 13.7)
- CKD after AKI (Table 13.8)

Table 13.5 CIN after PCI [14]

Variables	Score
Presentation	
Asymptomatic or stable angina	0
Unstable angina	2
NSTEMI	4
STEMI	8
eGFR	
≥60	0
30–59	1
<30	4
LV EF < 40%	2
DM	
No DM	0
No insulin	1
On insulin	2
Hb <11 g/dL	1
Basal glucose ≥150 mg/dL	1
CHF at presentation	1
Age > 75 years	1

Event Rate

Risk category	Score	AKI (%)
Low risk	≤2	0.6
Moderate	3–7	2.4
High	8–11	11.5
Very high	12≤	33.7

Prevention Protocol [15]

Category	eGFR>60 ml/min per 1.73 m2	No DM/HF with eGFR 30–60 DM/HF with eGFR 45–60	No DM/HF with eGFR <30 DM/HF with eGFR <45 or Monoclonal gammapathy
Strategy	Leveral fluid intake 1 L over 12 h before and after contrast	Oral volume expansion schedule 1 gNaCl +150 mL of water every hour for 2 h before until 6 h after contrast	IV volume expansion with NS or sodium bicarbonate 1 L NS over 12 h before and after the contrast Or 1 L of D5 + 150 mmol/L bicarbonate 8.4%/L, 3 mL/kg/hr. over 1 h before and 1 mL/kg/hr. for 6 h after contrast

Table 13.6 Rhabdomyolysis [16]

Variables	Score
Age	
50 < to ≤70	1.5
70 < to ≤80	2.5
80<	3
Female sex	1
Initial creatinine mg/dL	
1.4–2.2	1.5
2.2<	3
Initial calcium <7.5 mg/dL	2
Initial CPK > 40,000 U/L	2
Origin not seizures, syncope, exercise, statin or myositis	3
Initial phosphate mg/dL	
4.0–5.4	1.5
5.4<	3
Initial bicarbonate <19 mEq/L	2

Risk category (score)	In-hospital mortality or RRT (%)
Low (<5)	1.2
Intermediate (5–10)	17.4
High (10<)	59.9

Table 13.7 Prediction of worsening renal function with HF admission "Forman Rule" [17]

Risk factors	Score
Hx of prior CHF	1
DM	1
SBP > 160	1
1.5 ≤ creatinine<2.5	2
2.5 ≤ creatinine	3

Score	Likelihood of developing worsening of renal function in the study group	Relative Risk for developing worsening of renal function
0	9.8%	1 (reference)
1	18.7%	1.91
2	20.3%	2.08
3	30.3%	3.11
4+	52.8%	5.40

Table 13.8 CKD after AKI [18]

6-variable and scores	
1. Age	
Age	Points
<50	0
50–59	1
60–69	2
70–79	2
80–89	2
90≤	3
2. Sex	
Sex	Points
Men	0
Women	3
3. Baseline Scr (mgldL)	
Scr mg/dL	Points
<0.6	0
0.6– < 0.7	1
0.7– < 0.8	1
0.8– < 0.9	2
0.9– < 1.0	2
1.0– < 1.1	3
1.1– < 1.2	3
1.2– < 1.3	4
1.3≤	5

4. Albuminemia			
Category	ACR	UA protein	Points
Normal	≤ 30 mg/g	Negative	0
Mild	30–300 mg/g	1+	1
Heavy	300 <	2+ ≤	3
Not measured	–	–	1

5. AKI		
Stage	criteria	Points
1	Cr increase ≥0.3 mg/dL or > × 1.5–1.9 times of baseline	0
2	Cr increase × 2.0–2.9 times of baseline	1
3	Cr increase ≥ × 3.0 times of baseline or increase ≥4.0 mg/dL	3

6. Discharge Scr (mg/dL)	
Scr (mg/dL)	Points
<1.0	0
1.0– < 1.3	3
1.3– < 1.6	6
1.6– < 1.9	7
1.9≤	11

Outcome

Points	Predicted risk of advanced CKD (%)
1–8	<1
9–14	1– < 5
15–17	5– < 10
18–19	10– < 20
20≤	20≤

References

1. Mercado M, et al. Acute kidney injury: diagnosis and management. AFP. 2019;100(11):687–94.
2. ☺☺Moore P, et al. Management of acute kidney injury: core curriculum 2018. Am J Kidney Dis. 2018;72(1):136–48.
3. Pannu N, Nadim M. An overview of drug-induced acute kidney injury. Crit Care Med. 2008;36(Suppl):S216–23.
4. Kulvichit W, et al. Biomarkers in acute kidney injury. Crit Care Clin. 2021;37:385–98.
5. Ostermann M, Joannidis M. Acute kidney injury 2016: diagnosis and diagnostic workup. Crtical Care. 2016;20:299. https://doi.org/10.1186/s13054-016-1478-z.
6. Belcher J, et al. Clinical applications of biomarkers for acute kidney injury. Am J Kidney Dis. 2011;57(6):930–40.
7. Ronco C, et al. Acute kidney injury. Lancet. 2019;394:1949–64.
8. Levey A, et al. National kidney foundation practice guidelines for chronic kidney disease: evaluation, classification, and stratification. Ann Intern Med. 2003;139:137–47.
9. ☺☺Stevens L, et al. Assessing kidney function-measured and estimated glomerular filtration rate. N Engl J Med. 2006;354:2473–83.
10. ☺☺☺Sethi S, et al. Acute glomerulonephritis. Lancet. 2022;399:1646–63.
11. ☺Lameire N, et al. Acute renal failure. Lancet. 2005;365:417–30.
12. ☺☺☺Darmon M, et al. Diagnostic work-up and specific causes of acute kidney injury. Intensive Care Med. 2017;43:829–40.
13. Moledina D, Perazella M. Drug-induced acute interstitial nephritis. Clin J Am Soc Nephrol. 2017;12:2046–9.
14. Mehran R, et al. A contemporary simple risk score for prediction of contract-associated acute kidney injury after percutaneous coronary interventions: derivation and validation from an observational registry. Lancet. 2021;398:1974–83.
15. Vanmassenhove J, et al. Intensive care medicine and renal transplantation 1. Management of patients at risk of acute kidney injury. Ibid. 2017;389:2139–51.
16. McMahon G, et al. A risk prediction score for kidney failure or mortality in rhabdomyolysis. JAMA Intern Med. 2013;173(19):1821–8.
17. Forman D, et al. Incidence, predictors at admission, and impact of worsening renal function among patients hospitalized with heart failure. J Am Coll Cardiol. 2004;43:61–7.
18. James M, et al. Derivation and external validation of prediction models for advanced chronic kidney disease following acute kidney injury. JAMA. 2017;318(18):1787–97.

Diuretics

14

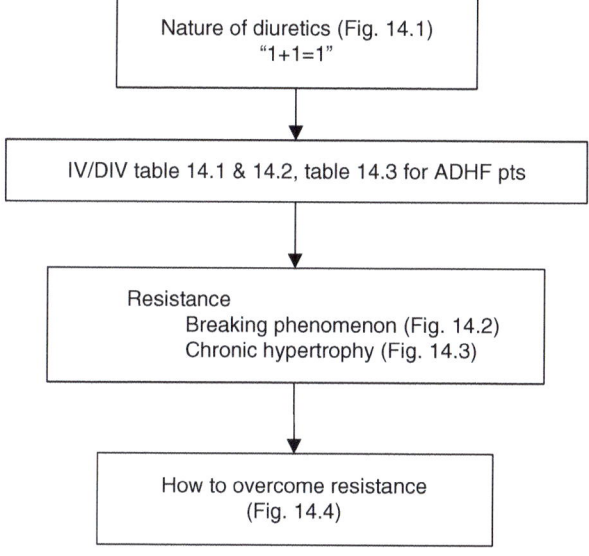

- "1 + 1 = 1" [1–3]
- All diuretics other than spironolactone works from the lumen of the nephron [2]

© The Author(s), under exclusive license to Springer Nature Switzerland AG 2025
M. J. Morikawa, *The Inpatient Medicine Handbook*,
https://doi.org/10.1007/978-3-032-08398-2_14

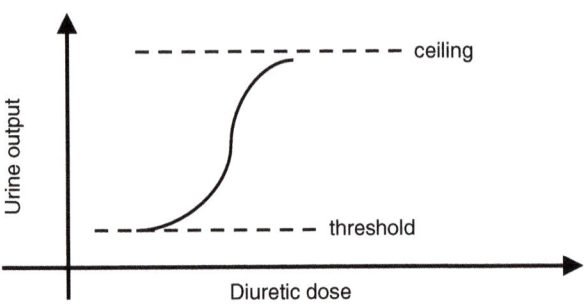

Fig. 14.1 Diuretics dynamics

Diuretics Strategies [1–3]

Table 14.1 IV dose

• Ceiling dose IV of diuretics (mg)					
	Moderate renal insufficiency	Severe insufficiency	Nephrotic syndrome	LC	CHF
Furosemide	80–160	160–200	80–120	40	40–80
Bumetanide	4–8	8–10	2–3	1	1–2
Torsemide	20–50	50–100	20–50	10	10–20

Table 14.2 DIV table

• Continuous infusion (DIV) (mg)				
	Loading dose	CCr < 25 (mL/min)	25–75	75<
Furosemide	40	20 then 40	10 then 20	10
Bumetanide	1	1 then 2	0.5 then 1	0.5
Torsemide	20	10 then 20	5 then 10	5

- There are two ways to dose diuretics: urine output strategy vs urine sodium strategy [4]
- For ADHF patient, try stepwise doing regimen [3, 5–7]

Table 14.3 ADHF DIV table

Furosemide			Metolazone
Previous oral dose (mg)	Bolus (mg)	DIV rate (mg/h)	Oral dose (mg)
≤80	40	5	NA
81–160	80	10	5 QD
161–240	80	20	5 BID
240 <	80	30	5 BID

Diuretic Resistance

- Two different types of resistance: acute (braking phenomenon) and chronic (hypertrophy of distal nephron segments [2, 3])

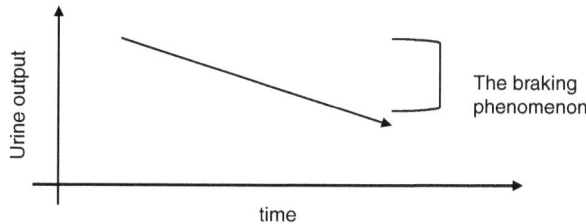

Fig. 14.2 Breaking phenomenon

"hypertrophy of DCT" after chronic loop use [8]

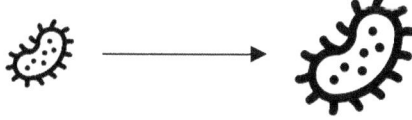

Fig. 14.3 Chronic hypertrophy of the cell

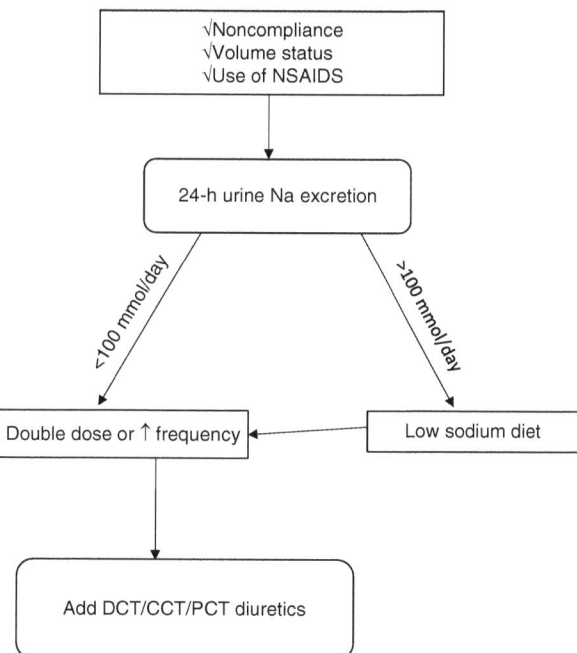

Fig. 14.4 For diuretic resistance
Based on Hoorn and Zietse [9]

References

1. Brater D. Diuretic therapy. N Engl J Med. 1998;339:387–95.
2. Brater D. Update in diuretic therapy: clinical pharmacology. Semin Nephrol. 2011;31:483–94.
3. ☺☺☺Ellison D, Felker G. Diuretic treatment in heart failure. N Engl J Med. 2017;377:1964–75.
4. Felker M, et al. Diuretic therapy for patients with heart failure. J Am Coll Cardiol. 2020;75:1178–95.
5. Grodin J, et al. Intensification of medication therapy for cardiorenal syndrome in acute decompensated heart failure. J Cardiac Fail. 2016;22(1):26–32.
6. ☺Ellison D. Clinical pharmacology in diuretic use. Clin J Am Soc Nephrol. 2019;14:1248–57.
7. ☺ ☺Jentzer J, et al. Contemporary management of severe acute kidney injury and refractory cardiorenal syndrome. J Am Coll Cardiol. 2020;76:1084–101.
8. ☺ ☺Subramanya A, Ellison D. Distal convoluted tubule. Clin J Am Soc Nephrol. 2014;9:2147–63.
9. Hoorn E, Zietse R. Diagnosis and treatment of hyponatremia: compilation of the guidelines. J Am Soc Nephrol. 2017;28:1340–9.

Anemia

15

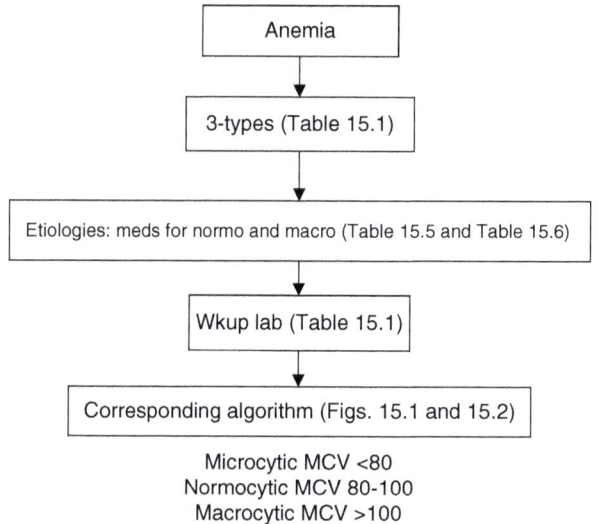

Microcytic MCV <80
Normocytic MCV 80-100
Macrocytic MCV >100

Table 15.1 3 categories of anemia

	Microcytic	Normocytic	Macrocytic
Etiologies	AI, IDA, thalassemia, sideroblastic [1]	Nutritional (IDA VitB12), hemolytic, renal insufficiency, bleeding [2]	Drugs, Vit B12, ETOH, MDS [3]
Wkup	Ferritin, Hb elecropheresis, Hepcidin, sTr/ferritin	Hemolysis lab (haptoglobin, LDH, indirect bilirubin, retic count) PBS, renal function, Coag DAT	Reticulocyte, PBS, B12, MMA, homocysteine

M. J. Morikawa, *The Inpatient Medicine Handbook*,
https://doi.org/10.1007/978-3-032-08398-2_15

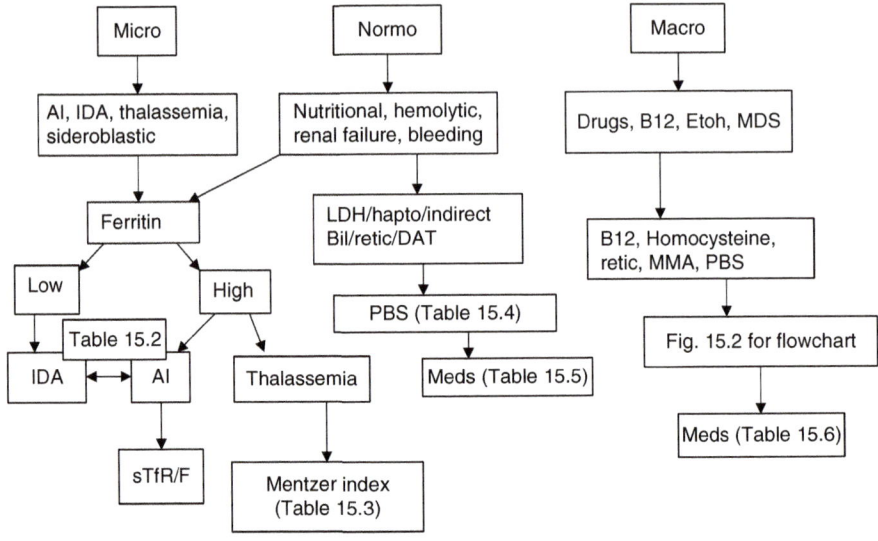

Fig. 15.1 Workup

Microcytic anemia
- Ferritin <15 diagnostic for IDA older than 5 years old [4]
- Ferritin >100 r/o IDA [5, 6]

IDA vs IA

- Serum soluble transferrin receptors (sTfR) inversely related to iron storage and not affected by inflammation [4, 7])
- Hepcidin production decreases in IDA but increase in AI [4]
- sTr/ferritin ratio help AI vs IDA in the elderly [7–10]

Table 15.2 IAD vs AI

	sTfR	Hepcidin	sTfR/Ferritin
IDA	↑	↓	>1.5
AI	→	↑	< 1

Follow the process below

1. Ferritin <30 ng/ml then IDA
2. Ferritin >100 ng/ml then most likely AI
3. Ferritin 30–100 then obtain sTfR

4. sTfR/log ferritin <1 then AI
5. sTfR/log ferritin >2 then AI + IDA
(Lanier et al.[8]; Weiss and Goodnough [9])

Thalassemia Mentzer index < 13 [11].

Table 15.3 Mentzer index: MCV/RBC count

	IDA	Thalassemia
RDW	high	Normal
Ferritin	low	Normal
Mentzer index	>13	<13

Normocytic

- Bleeding, renal disease, hemolysis, and nutritional
- Hapto, LDH, indirect Bil, retic, PBS, DAT (direct Coombs test)

Table 15.4 Peripheral blood smear (PBS)

cells	Diagnosis
schistocyte	TMA (HUS, TTP, HITT, HELLP)
Sickle cell	SCD
Bite cell, Heinz body	G6PD def
Spherocyte	DAT - hereditary spherocytosis
	DAT + autoimmune hemolytic anemia
Elliptocyte	Hereditary elliptocytosis

DAT direct antiglobulin test
(Based on Dhaliwal et al. [12]; Phillips and Henderson [13])

Table 15.5 Meds

Mechanism	Medications
Drug induced AIHA	Methyldopa, penicillin
	Cefotetan, ceftriaxone, piperacillin, zosyn, NSAIDs
Drug induced TMA	Quinine, cyclosporine, tacrolimus and others
Oxidative hemolysis in G6PD	Nitrofurantoin
	Phenazopyridine
	Rifampin
	ribavirin

(Dhaliwal et al. [12]; Phillip and Henderson [13])

Macrocytic Anemia

- 4 conditions: Etoh, Drug, Vit B, MDS,
- PBS, retic count
- MMA (methylmalonic acid), homocysteine, Vit B12

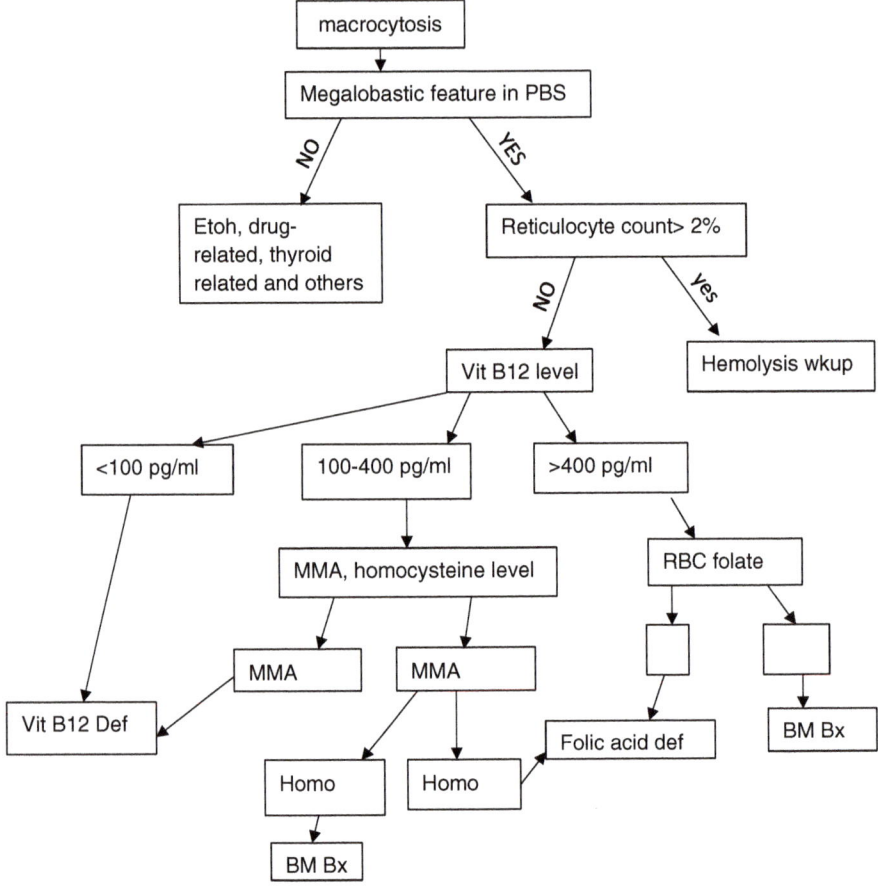

Fig. 15.2 For macrocytosis.(Based on Kaferle and Strzoda [3]; Langan and Goodbred [14])

Table 15.6 Meds

category	Meds
Reverse transcriptase inhibitors (HIV tx)	Stavudine, lamivudine, zidovudine
Anticonvulsants	Valproic acid, phenytoin
Folate antagonist	Methotrexate
Chemotherapeutics	Alkylating agents, pyrimidine, purine inhibitors
Others	Trimethoprim/sulfamethoxazole Biguanides

(Based on Kaferle and Strzoda [3])

References

1. DeLoughery T. Microcytic anemia. N Engl J Med. 2014;371:1324–31.
2. ☺☺☺Tefferi A. How to interpret and pursue an abnormal complete blood cell count in adults. Mayo Clin Proc. 2005;80:923–36.
3. Kaferle J, Strzoda C. Evaluation of macrocytosis. AFP. 2009;79:203–8.
4. Lopez A, et al. Iron deficiency anemia. Lancet. 2016;387:907–16.
5. Killip S, et al. Iron deficiency anemia. AFP. 2007;75:671–8.
6. Van Vranken M. Evaluation of microcytosis. Ibid. 2010;82(9):1117–22.
7. ☺☺☺Ganz T. Anemia of inflammation. N Engl J Med. 2019;381:1148–57.
8. Lanier J, et al. Anemia in older adults. AFP. 2018;98(7):437–42.
9. Weiss G, Goodnough L. Anemia of chronic disease. In: N Engl J Med, vol. 352; 2005. p. 1011–23.
10. Rimon E, et al. Diagnosis of iron deficiency anemia in the elderly by transferrin receptor-ferritin index. Arch Intern Med. 2002;162:445–9.
11. Muncie H, Campbell J. Alpha and Beta thalassemia. AFP. 2009;80(4):339–44.
12. ☺☺☺Dhaliwal G, et al. Hemolytic anemia. Ibid. 2004;69(11):2599–606.
13. ☺Phillips J, Henderson A. Hemolytic anemia: evaluation and differential diagnosis. Ibid. 2018;98(6):354–61.
14. Langan R, Goodbred A. Vitamin B12 deficiency: recognition and management. Ibid. 2017;96:384–9.

Thrombocytopenia

16

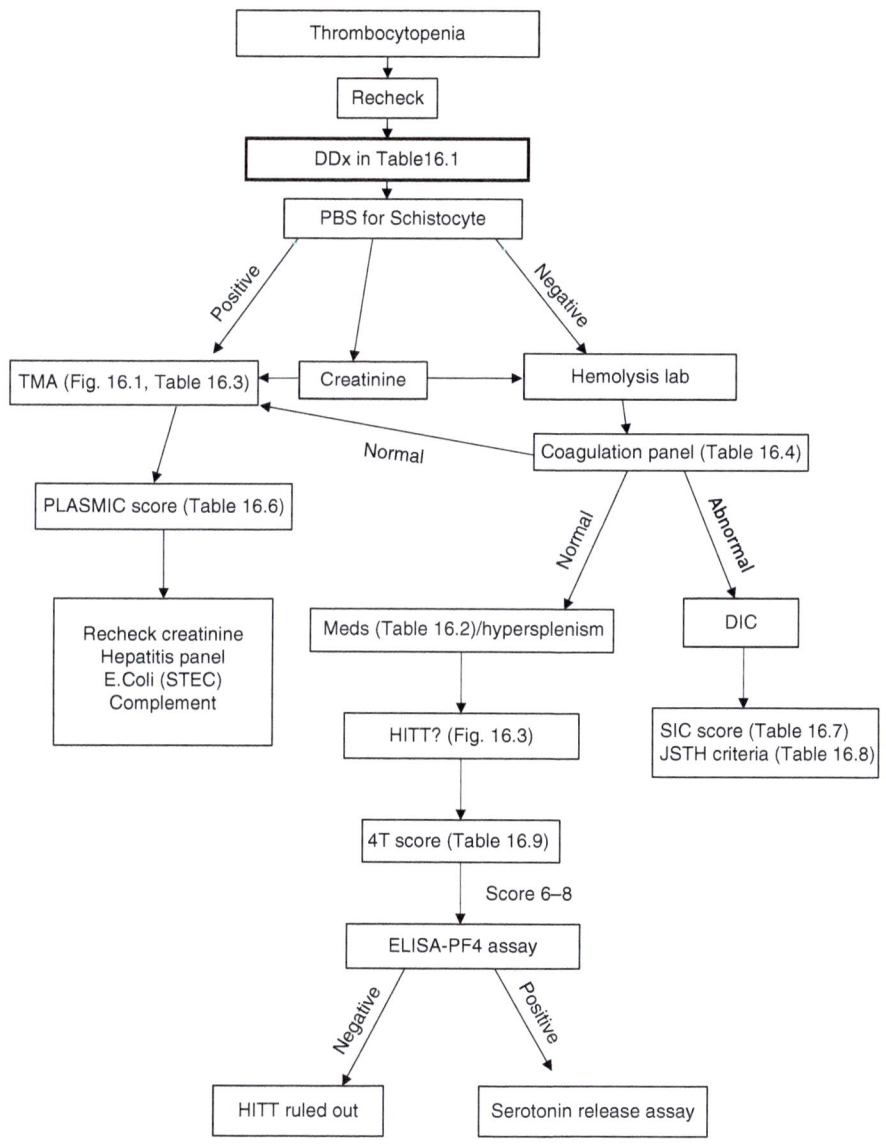

General:

Three most common causes of thrombocytopenia in inpatient service:

1. Infection
2. Medication
3. Immunothrombocytopenia

Two medical conditions often associated with thrombocytopenia

1. LC
2. ESRD

Difference Between Platelet Disorder Versus Coagulation Disorder

	Platelet/vascular wall disorder	Coagulation disorder
Mucosal bleeding	+	−
Petechiae	+	−
Joint /deep hematomas	−	+

Based on Hoffbrand and Steensma [1]; Nackman and Rafii [2]

Table 16.1 DDx for thrombocytopenia before you consider TMA, HITT, ITP, DIC or HELLP

Lab error		
	Pseudothrombocytopenia	Recheck lab right away
Medical conditions		
	Renal and liver disease	LFT, Chem basic
Hematologic condition		
	Myelodysplastic syndrome, acute leukemia	Blood smear, BM
	Lymphoprolifeverative dis	BM
	Aplastic anemia	BM
	Genetic disease e.g. Bernard-Soulier syndrome	
	Evans syndrome (thrombocytopenia + direct antiglobulin + hemolytic anemia)	Blood smear, haptoglobin, LDH
	Immunothrombosis	See below for references
Infection		
	HIV, hepatitis, CMV, EBV, H pylori	Serologic PCR
Autoimmune disease		
	SLE, RA, APLS	ANA, RA, ACCPA, antiphospholipid ab
Meds	Table 16.2 below	

Based on Cooper and Ghanima [3]

Immunothrombosis:

- Platelet is an immune cell [4]
- Platelet-endothelial cross-talk via complement [5]
- Platelet—neutrophil (inflammation)—endothelium [6]

Table 16.2 Medications causing thrombocytopenia

• Typically needs 5–7 days of exposure to sensitize to the meds	
Categories	Meds
Heparins	UFH, LMWH
Cinchona alkaloids	Quinine, quinidine
Platelet inhibitors	Abciximab, eptifibatide, tirofiban
Antirheumatics	Gold salts, D-penicillamine
Antimicrobials	Linezolid, rifampin, sulfonamides, vancomycin
Anticonvulsive	Carbamazepine, phenytoin, valproic acid, diazepam
H2 blocker	Cimetidine, ranitidine
Analgesics	Acetaminophen, diclofenac, naproxen, ibuprofen
Diuretics	HCTZ
Chemotherapneutic agents	Fludarabine, cyclosporine, rituximab

Based on Aster and Bougie [7]; Gauer and Braun [8]

TMA: Triad = thrombocytopenia; MAHA, and organ damage

Thrombotic microangiopathies (TMA) are groups of disorders characterized by (1) thrombocytopenia; (2) MAHA; and (3) organ dysfunction (e.g. AKI) [9, 10]

Fig. 16.1 Classification of TMA [9–11]

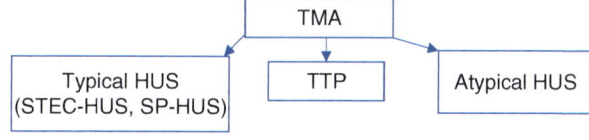

Table 16.3 TMA lab

Lab	
Schistocytes	Present in PBS
Haptoglobin	Reduction
Direct antiglobulin (Coombs) test (DAT)	Negative
Coagulation panel	Within normal limits

Azoulay et al. [10]; Manrique-Caballero et al. [11]

Fig. 16.2 DDx DIC,
TTP, HUS

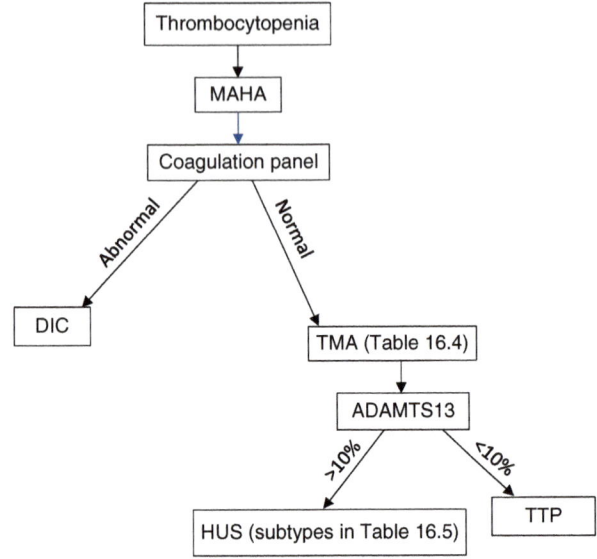

Table 16.4 DDx of TMA lab values

	Plt	MAHA	PT	PTT	Fibrinogen	ADAMTS13
TTP	↓	+	–	–	–	↓
HUS	↓	+	–	–	–	–
DIC	↓	+	↑	↑	↓	–

Manrique-Caballero et al. [11]

- TMA: imbalance between the platelet count and coagulation biomarkers, PT and
  D-dimer changes are usually moderate to mild in TMA [12]

Table 16.5 HUS subtypes

	Coombs test	Stool PCR
SP-HUS (S pneumoniae HUS)	+	–
STEC-HUS (Shiga toxin associated HUS)	–	+
aHUS (atypical HUS)	–	–

Table 16.6 PLASMIC score

• Score to identify patients with ADAMATS 13 <10%
Underlying features
  No active cancer
  No hx of BM or solid organ transplant
Laboratory parameters
  Platelet <30,000/µL
  MCV <90
  Creatinine <20.0 mg/dL
  INR <1.5
  Hemolysis (either reticulocyte >2.5%, indirect bilirubin >2.0 mg/dL or absent haptoglobin)

Proportion ADAMATS13 ≤10%	
Risk category	%
Low (0–4)	4.3
Intermediate (5–6)	56.8
High (7)	96.2

Bendapudi et al. [13]; Phillip and Henderson [14]

DIC:

• Systememic activation of coagulation causes thrombosis and bleeding at the same time [15]
• Diverse causes [15]

  Sepsis
  Trauma
  Cancer
  OB complication
  Vascular disorder
  Toxins
  Immunologic disorders

• No single test can diagnose DIC
• Impaired fibrinolysis caused by activation of PAI-1 [12, 15]
• Microthrombi in sepsis is caused by immunothrombus [12]

Table 16.7 Sepsis-induced coagulopathy (SIC) score

Variable	Points
INR	
≤1.2	0
1.2<	1
1.4<	2
Platelet (×10⁹/L)	
≥150	0
<150	1
<100	2
SOFA four items	
0	0
1	1
2≤	2

- SOFA four item is the sum of respiratory SOFA, CVD SOFA, hepatic SOFA and renal SOFA
- SIC score ≥4 had more than 20% mortality.

Iba et al. [16]

Table 16.8 JSTH DIC criteria

- Three categories of DIC, hematopoietic type omitted the platelet count score, infectious type omitted the fibrinogen score and basic type based on the underlying pathology.
- The combination of global coagulation tests with HMMs (hemostatic molecular markers) had the highest ARC values.
- Global coagulation tests:
    Platelet count, Prothrombin time (PT), fibrinogen and fibrin-related markers
- Hemostatic molecular markers (HMMs)
    Antithrombin (AT) activity
    Soluble fibrin (SF)
    Thrombin AT complex (TAT), prothrombin complex F1 + 2(F1 + 2)

	Basic	Hematopoietic	Infectious
GCT			
Platelet			
>120	0		0
80<–≤120	1		1
50<–≤80	2		2
≤50	3		3
FDP (fibrin degradation product)			
<10	0	0	0
10≤–<20	1	1	1
20≤–<40	2	2	2
≥40	3	3	3
Fibrinogen (mg/dL)			
>150	0	0	
100<–≤150	1	1	
≤100	2	2	
PT			
<1.25	0	0	0
1.25≤–<1.67	1	1	1
≥1.67	2	2	2
HMMs			
Antithrombin (%)			
>70	0	0	0
≤70	1	1	1
TAT, SF or F1 + 2			
<x2 of NUL	0	0	0
≥x2 of NUL	1	1	1
Liver failure			
No	0	0	0
Yes	−3	−3	−3

- DIC diagnosis

Basic	Hematopoietic	Infectious
≥6	≥4	≥5

Wada et al. [17]

HIT:

- The incidence is x10 times higher among UFH exposure than among LMWH [18]

Table 16.9 4T score

	0	1	2
Thrombocytopenia	Decrease <30% or nadir ≤10,000	Decrease 30–50% or nadir 10,000–19,000	Decrease >50% and nadir ≥20,000
Timing of onset	≤4 days with no recent heparin exposure	>10 days or unclear exposure	5–10 days or day 1 if recent exposure
Thrombosis	None	Progressive or recurrent thrombosis	New thrombosis or anaphylactoid reaction after heparin bolus
Other causes of thrombocytopenia	Definite	Possible	None

Risk category	Score
low	0–3
intermediate	4–5
High	6–8

- Total score <4 has very high NPV, whereas high score (6–8) has high PPV

Lo et al. [19]; Greinacher [18]; Kalpatthi and Kiss [20]; Menajovsky [21]

Table 16.10 Tx for HITT

	Clearance	Half-life	Monitoring
Argatroban	Hepatobiliary	40–50 min	aPTT
Bivalirudin	Renal	25 min	aPTT
Fondaparinux	Renal	17–20 h	None
Desirudin	Renal	2–3 h	None
Danaparoid	Renal	24 h	Anti-Xa activity

Based on Kelton et al. [22]

- Bivalirudin protocol for CPB [23]
- Anti-PF4/heparin Ab level correlates with 30-day risk of PE and thrombosis [24]

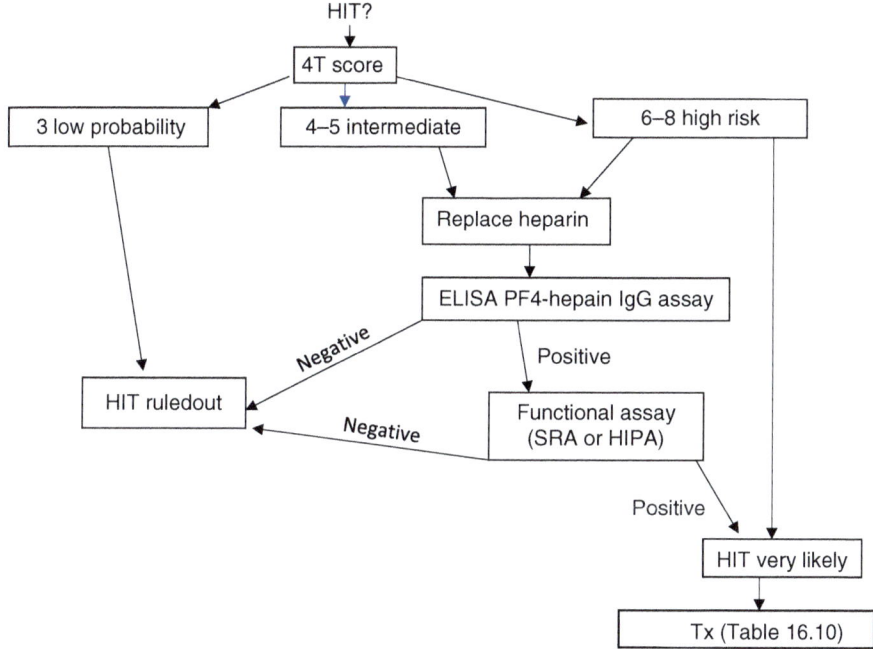

Fig. 16.3 Algorithm for HIT [18, 20]

ITP

- Plt <100,000 if other causes are r/o [25]
- 2 peaks in incidence: 20–30 and 60<

References

1. Hoffbrand A, Steensma D. Hoffbrand's essential haematology. Hoboken: John Wiley & Sons; 2020.
2. ☺ ☺ Nachman R, Rafii S. Platelets, petechiae, and preservation of the vascular wall. N Engl J Med. 2008;359:1261–70.
3. ☺ Cooper N, Ghanima W. Immune thrombocytopenia. N Engl J Med. 2019;381:945–55.
4. ☺ ☺ McFadyen J, Kaplan Z. Platelets are not just for clots. Transfusion Med Rev. 2015;29:110–9.
5. ☺ van der Poll T, Parker R. Platelet activation and endothelial cell dysfunction. Crit Care Clin. 2020;36:233–53.
6. Li J, et al. Platelet-neutrophil interactions under thromboinflammatory conditions. Cell Mol Life Sci. 2015;72:2627–43.
7. ☺ Aster R, Bougie D. Drug-induced immune thrombocytopenia. N Engl J Med. 2007;357:580–7.
8. Gauer R, Braun M. Thrombocytopenia. AFP. 2012;85(6):612–22.
9. ☺ George J, Nester C. Syndromes of thrombotic microangiopathy. N Engl J Med. 2014;371:654–66.

10. ☺ ☺ Azoulay E, et al. Expert statement on the standard of care in critically ill adult patients with atypical hemolytic uremic syndrome. Chest. 2017;152(2):424–34.
11. Manrique-Caballero C, et al. Typical and atypical hemolytic uremic syndrome in the critically ill. Crit Care Clin. 2020;36:333–56.
12. Iba T, et al. Roles of coagulation abnormalities and microthrombosis in sepsis: pathophysiology, diagnosis and treatment. Arch Med Res. 2021;52:788–97.
13. Bendapudi P, et al. Derivation and prospective validation of a predictive score for the rapid diagnosis of thrombotic thrombocytopenic purpura: the plasmic score. Blood. 2014;124(21):231.
14. Phillips J, Henderson A. Hemolytic anemia: evaluation and differential diagnosis. AFP. 2018;98(6):354–61.
15. Levi M, Ten Cate H. Disseminated intravascular coagulation. N Engl J Med. 1999;341:586–92.
16. Iba T, et al. New criteria for sepsis-induced coagulopathy (SIC) following the revised sepsis definition: a retrospective analysis of a nationwide survey. BMJ Open. 2017;7:e017046. https://doi.org/10.1136/bmjopen-2017;017046.
17. Wada H, et al. The approval of revised diagnostic criteria for DIC from the Japanese Society on Thrombosis and Hemostasis. Thromb J. 2017;15:17. https://doi.org/10.1186/s12959-017-0142-4.
18. ☺ ☺ ☺ Greinacher A. Heparin-induced thrombocytopenia. N Engl J Med. 2015;373:252–61.
19. Lo G, et al. Evaluation of pretest clinical score (4 T's) for the diagnosis of heprain-induced thrombocytopenia in two clinical settings. J Thromb Haemost. 2006;4:759–65.
20. Kalpatthi R, Kiss J. Thrombotic thrombocytopenic purpura, heparin-induced thrombocytopenia, and disseminated intravascular coagulation. Crit Care Clin. 2020;36:357–77.
21. Menajovsky L. Heparin-induced thrombocytopenia: clinical manifestations and management strategies. Am J Med. 2005;118:215–305.
22. ☺ Kelton J, et al. Nonheparin anticoagulants for heparin-induced thrombocytopenia. N Engl J Med. 2013;368:737–44.
23. Salter B, et al. Heparin-induced thrombocytopenia. J Am Coll Cardiol. 2016;67(21):2519–32.
24. Baroletti S, et al. Thrombosis in suspected haparin-induced thrombocytopenia occurs more often with high antibody levels. Am J Med. 2012;125:44–9.
25. ☺ ☺ Cooper N, Ghanima W. Immune thrombocytopenia. N Engl J Med. 2019;381:945–55.

Substance Abuse

17

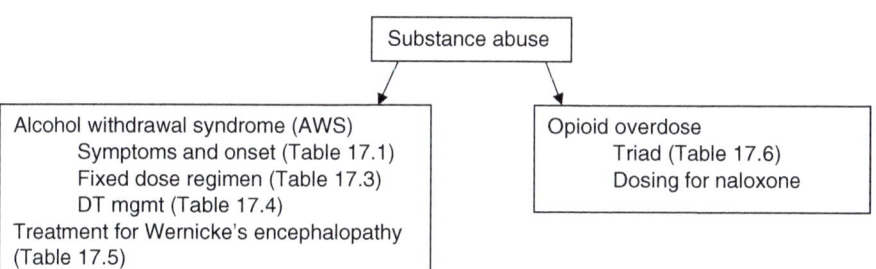

Alcohol withdrawal syndrome (AWS)

- Intermittent binge doesn't lead to AWS [1]
- Clinical stages and symptoms are classified into four categories either by symptoms or time of onset from cessation of alcohol but slightly different among authors: compare those classifications:
- Four clinical stages: autonomic hyperactivity; hallucination; neuronal excitation (seizures); and DT [2]
- Symptoms don't progress linearly from one stage to the next,
- Types and timing [3, table 1, fig 2, 4]
- Alcohol hallucination doesn't predict dT [2]
- CIWA is NOT validated in ICU [1]
- DT begins about 3 days after appearance of symptoms of alcohol withdrawal and lasts from 1 to 8 days [5]
- Approximately 5% of patients develop DT [2, 5]
- Approximately 1–4% of hospitalized pts with DT die [5]

© The Author(s), under exclusive license to Springer Nature Switzerland AG 2025
M. J. Morikawa, *The Inpatient Medicine Handbook*,
https://doi.org/10.1007/978-3-032-08398-2_17

Table 17.1 Alcohol related symptoms and timeline

Stages	Onset	Peak	Incidence	Symptoms
Uncomplicated withdrawal (Shakes)	8 h	24–36 h	80%	Minor tremor, N/V, tachycardia, irritability, HTN
Alcohol withdrawal seizure (Rum fits)	12 h; 24–48 h	12–48 h	5–15%	Tonic-clonic seizures
Alcohol hallucination	8 h: 12–24 h	24–96 h	Up to 30%	Visual/tactile hallucination
Alcohol withdrawal delirium (delirium tremens)	48–72 h	4–5 days	Up to 5%	Agitation, delirium, tremor

Based on Bayard et al. [4]; Schuckit [5]; Carlson et al. [1]; Maldonado [3]

MEDS

- Benzodiazepine (BZD) is the hallmark for AWS [6]
- BZD acts as GABA receptor agonists and functions as an alcohol replacement [2]
- No evidence that one BZD is better than another [5]
- For patients with LC, BZD not hepatically metabolized would be ideal, i.e. lorazepam or exazepam [2]
- Two different dosing is discussed in the literature: treatment for DT in ICU and inpatient/outpatient fixed dose/symptom-triggered regimen
- Fixed dose schedule uses does at specific interval regardless of symptoms [7]

Table 17.2 Medications

BZD	Routes	Dose	Half life	Comments
Chlordiapzepoxide	PO, IM, IV	25–50 mg	5–15 h	Long active metabolites
Diazepam	PO, IM, IV	10 mg	30–60 h	Early onset but long actii ng metabolites
Lorazepam	PO, IM, IV	2 mg	10–20 h	Intermediate half life (hepatic glucuronidation) less hepatotoxic
Carbamazepine	PO	600–800 mg	25 h	
Gabapentin	PO	300–600 mg	5–7 h	
Valpronic acid	PO	1000–1200 mg	9–16 h	

Modified from Maldonado [3]; Carlson et al. [1]; Muncie et al. [7]

Table 17.3 Lorazepam fixed dose regimen

2 mg PO Q6 × 24 h
2 mg PO Q8 × 24 h
1 mg PO Q8 × 24 h
1 mg Q12 × 24 h

Based on Muncie et al. [7]

Table 17.4 DT mgmt

Lorazepam 1–4 mg IV Q5–15 min, or 1–40 mg IM Q 30–60 min
Haldol 0.5–5 mg IV/IM Q30–60 min or 0.5–5 mg PO Q4 h
Thiamine 100 mg IV/IM × at least 3 days

Mayo-Smith et al. [8]; Schuckit [5]

Table 17.5 Tx for Wernicke's encephalopathy

Thiamine 500 mg IV × TID for 5 days

Schuckit [5]

Alternative agents other than BZD
Baclofen
Phenobarbital [1]
Carbamazepine/valproic acid [7]

Table 17.6 Triad of symptoms

Respiratory depression
Miosis
Stupor

Boyer [9]

Opioid Overdose

- If RR <12/min strongly suggest opioid overdose
- Naloxone IV onset of action <2 min and duration of action 20–90 min
- Naloxone 0.04 mg IV × one and repeat every 2 min with increasing dose as follows:

Q2–3 min
0.5 mg, 2 mg, 4 mg, 10 mg, then 15 mg

References

1. ☺ ☺ ☺ Carlson R, et al. Alcohol withdrawal syndrome. Crit Care Clin. 2012;28:549–85.
2. Sarff M, Gold J. Alcohol withdrawal syndromes in the intensive care unit. Crit Care Med. 2010;38(9 Suppl):S494–501.
3. Maldonado J. Novel algorithms for the prophylaxis and management of alcohol withdrawal syndromes- beyond benzodiazepines. Crit Care Clin. 2017;33:559–99.
4. Bayard M, et al. Alcohol withdrawal syndrome. Am Fam Physician. 2004;69:1443–50.

5. ☺ ☺ Schuckit M. Recognition and management of withdrawal delirium (Delirium Tremens). N Engl J Med. 2014;371:2109–13.
6. D'Onofrio G, et al. Lorazepam for the prevention of recurrent seizures related to alcohol. N Engl J Med. 1999;340:915–9.
7. Muncie H, et al. Outpatient management of alcohol withdrawal syndrome. Am Fam Physician. 2013;88(9):589–95.
8. Mayo-Smith M, et al. Management of alcohol withdrawal delirium. Arch Intern Med. 2004;164:1405–12.
9. ☺ ☺ ☺ Boyer E. Management of opioid analgesic overdose. N Engl J Med. 2012;367:146–55.

Part II

Surgical Topics

Perioperative Medicine 18

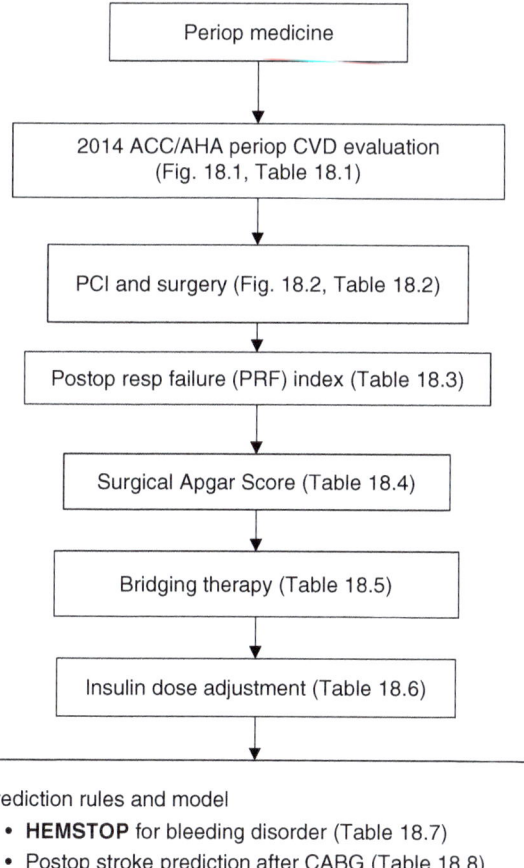

© The Author(s), under exclusive license to Springer Nature Switzerland AG 2025

M. J. Morikawa, *The Inpatient Medicine Handbook*,

https://doi.org/10.1007/978-3-032-08398-2_18

CVD Risk Stratification

- Upstream coronary revascularization didn't improve perioperative outcomes [1]
- High dose extended release metoprolol succinate (100 mg/day) initiate immediate before surgery is increased perioperative stroke and mortality
- Surgery should be delayed at least 30 days after BM stent and 12 months after DES.

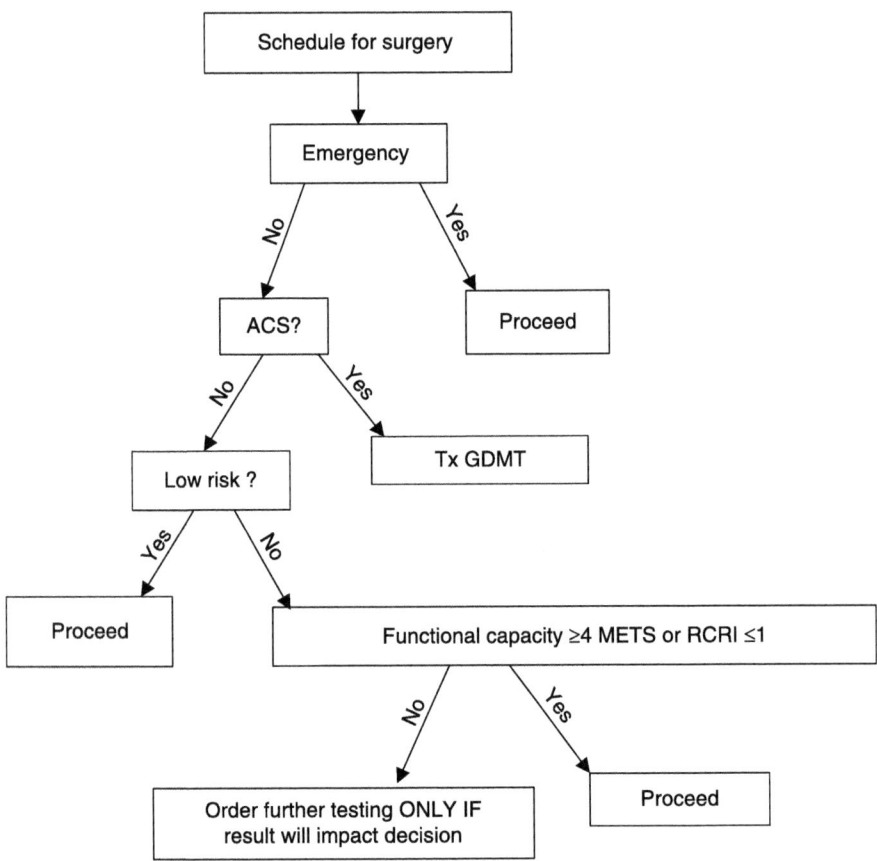

Fig. 18.1 Perioperative cardiac clearance

Surgery and MACE Risk

MACE risk	Types of surgery
<1% risk	Cataract surgery
	Cosmetic or plastic surgery
≥1% risk	Orthopedic surgery
	ENT surgery
	Urological surgery
≥3% risk	General abdominal or intraperitoneal surgery
	Neurosurgery
≥5% risk	Suprainguinal and peripheral vascular surgery
	Thoracic surgery
	Transplant surgery

Smilowitz and Berger [1]

Table 18.1 Revised Cardiac Risk Index (RCRI)

1. High-risk surgery
2. Ischemic heart disease
3. Hx of CHF
4. Hx of CVA
5. Insulin tx for DM
6. Preop creatinine >2.0 mg/dL

- High-risk type of surgery: Intraperitoneal, intrathoracic, or suprainguinal vascular procedures

Rate of major cardiac complications

Score	Outcome (%)
0	0.4
1	0.9
2	7
≥3	11

Lee et al. [2]

Table 18.2 Revascularization and surgery

CABG for	Wait at least 60 days and DAPT should be discontinued 5 days before surgery but
MI	ASA should be continued
BMS	Wait at least 30 days
DES	Wait at least 3 months (preferably 6 months)

Ganesh et al. [3]

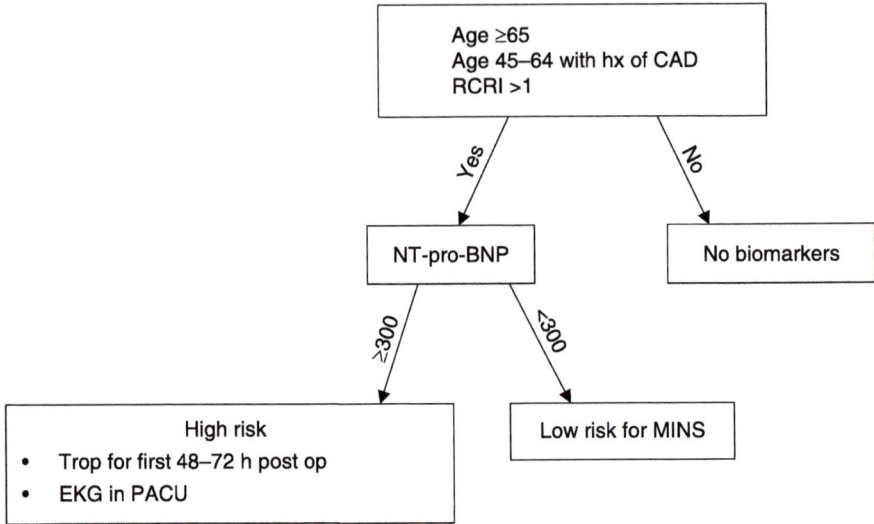

Fig. 18.2 Risk stratification by biomarkers for high risk patient for MI after noncardiac surgery (MINS) [3]

Periop Respiratory Complications

Table 18.3 Postoperative respiratory failure (PRF) index

• PRF: inability to extubate 48 h after surgery or unplanted intubation within 48 h	
Variable	Point
Type of surgery	
AAA	27
Thoracic	21
Neurosurgery, upper abdominal or PVD	14
Neck	11
Emergency surgery	11
Albumin <3.0 g/dL	9
BUN >30 mg/dL	8
Partially or fully dependent functional status	7
Hx of COPD	6
Age	
≥70	6
60–69	4

Outcome by class		
Class	Points	PRF rate (%)
1	≤10	0.5
2	11–19	1.8
3	20–27	4.2
4	28–40	10.1
5	40<	26.6

Arozullah et al. [4]

- Incentive spirometry and deep breathing exercise are the most beneficial modalities to prevent post-op pulmonary complications [5–7]

Table 18.4 Surgical Apgar

	Points				
Variable	0	1	2	3	4
EBL (ml)	>1000	601–1000	101–600	≤100	
Lowest MAP mmHg	<40	40–54	55–69	≥70	
Lowest HR/min	>85	76–85	66–75	56–65	≤55

- Bradyarrhythmia receives 0 points for lowest HR

30 days death rate

Score	0–2	3–4	5–6	7–8	9–10
Mortality (%)	44	16	5	2	0.1

Regenbogen et al. [8]

Bridging Therapy

- Balance between thromboembolic risk and post op bleeding risk
- Three conditions should be considered for thromboembolic risk (Af, VTE, and mechanical valve)

Table 18.5 For bridging therapy (BT)

	Estimated annual VTE rate	MV	VTE	Af
Low	<5%	Bileaflet aortic prosthetic valve without Af and no other risk for stroke	VTE >12 months previously and no other RFs	Non valvular Af with CHADS2 0–2 and no hx of CVA or TIA
Moderate	5–10	Bileaflet prosthetic aortic valve with ≥1 RFs Af Previous stroke or TIA HTN DM CHF Age >75	VTE 3–12 months Recurrent VTE Non-severe thrombophilia Active cancer	CHADS2 3–4
high	>10	Any mitral prosthetic valve Any cagd-ball or tilting disc aortic prosthetic valve Recent (<6 months) stroke or TIA	Recent (<3 months) VTE Severe thrombophilia	CHADS2 score 5–6 Rheumatic VHD Recent (<3 months) hx of stroke or TIA

Based on Daniel [9]; Baron et al. [10]

- Indication for BT

MV	VTE	Af
Bileaflet Aortic valve with no other risk is the only condition for **no** BT	VTE <3 months or severe thrombophilia	CHADS2 ≥4 or prior CVA or cardiac thrombus

Baron et al. [10]

- When to resume bridging therapy is depending on bleeding risk of procedure: non-high risk: resume 24 h after the procedure, and high bleeding risk, then resume 48–72 h after the procedure [9]

Table 18.6 Perioperative Insulin adjustment

• Insulin doses for periop in T2DM		
Insulin type	Night before surgery	Morning of surgery
Long-acting (glargine, detemir)	75–80% dose	50% dose
NPH	75–80% dose	50% dose
Regular Rapid-acting	Normal dose	Withhold
Pump	Normal dose	60–80% normal base rate and withhold short-acting

Himes et al. [11]

Table 18.7 HEMSTOP questions to identify bleeding disorders

- Score ≥2 had Sensitivity 89% and specificity of 98.6% for bleeding disorder
1. Have you ever consulted a doctor or received tx for prolonged or unusual bleeding?
2. Do you experience burises/hematomas >2 cm without trauma or severe bruising after minor trauma?
3. After a tooth extraction, have you ever experienced prolonged bleeding requiring medical/dental consultation?
4. Have you experienced excessive bleeding during or after surgery?
5. Is there anyone in your family who suffers from a coagulation disease?
For females:
6. Have you ever consulted a doctor or received a tx for heavy or prolonged menstrual periods?
7. Did you experience prolonged or excessive bleeding after delivery?

Bonhomme et al. [12]

Table 18.8 Post-op stroke prediction after CABG

Variable	Points
Age	
55–59	1.5
60–64	2.5
65–69	3.5
70–74	4
75–79	4.5
≥80	5.5
Female	1
DM	1.5
Vascular disease	2
Renal failure or Creatinine ≥2 mg/dl	2
EF <40%	1.5
Surgery	
Urgent	1.5
Emergent	2.5

Charlesworth et al. [13]

- Score ≥10 had >5% risk of stroke risk.

Table 18.9 Post-op delirium prediction rule

Risk factor	Points
Age ≥70	1
Alcohol abuse	1
Hx of cognitive impairment	1
Severe physical impairment (SAS class IV)	1
Na: <130 or >150; K <3.0 or >6.0; glucose <60 or >300 mg/dL	1
Aortic aneurysm surgery	2
Noncardiac thoracic surgery	1

Outcome	
Total points	Risk of delirium %
0	2
1–2	11
≥3	50

Marcantonio et al. [14]

References

1. ☺ ☺ ☺ Smilowitz N, Berger J. Perioperative cardiovascular risk assessment and management for noncardiac surgery. A review. JAMA. 2020;324(3):279–90.
2. Lee T, et al. Derivation and prospective validation of a simple index for prediction of cardiac risk of major noncardiac surgery. Circulation. 1999;100:1043–9.
3. ☺ ☺ ☺ Ganesh R, et al. Perioperative cardiac risk reduction in noncardiac surgery. Mayo Clin Proc. 2021;96(8):2260–76.
4. Arozullah A, et al. Multifactorial risk index for predicting postoperative respiratory failure in men after major noncardiac surgery. Ann Surg. 2000;232:242–53.

5. Westerdahl E, et al. Deep-breathing exercise reduce atelectasis and improve pulmonary function after coronary artery bypass surgery. Chest. 2005;128:3482–8.
6. Smetana G. A 68-year-old man with COPD contemplating colon cancer surgery. JAMA. 2007;297:2121–30.
7. Eltorai A, et al. Effect of an incentive spirometer patient reminder after coronary artery bypass grafting. A randomized clinical trial. JAMA Surg. 2019;154(7):579–88.
8. Regenbogen S, et al. Utility of the surgical apgar score. Validation in 4119 patients. Arch Surg. 2009;144:30–6.
9. ☺☺☺Daniels P. Peri-procedural management of patients taking oral anticoagulants. BMJ. 2015;351:h2391.
10. ☺☺☺Baron T, et al. Management of antithrombotic therapy in patients undergoing invasive procedures. N Engl J Med. 2013;368:2113–24.
11. Himes C, et al. Perioperative evaluation and management of endocrine disorders. Mayo Clin Proc. 2020;95(12):2760–74.
12. Bonhomme F, et al. Preoperative hemostatic assessment: a new and simple bleeding questionnaire. Can J Anesth. 2016;63:1007–15.
13. Charlesworth D, et al. Development and validation of a prediction model for strokes after coronary artery bypass grafting. Ann Thorac Surg. 2003;76:436–43.
14. Marcantonio E, et al. A clinical prediction rule for delirium after elective noncardiac surgery. JAMA. 1994;271:134–9.

Urinary Retention/Incontinence/Diversion

19

Retention

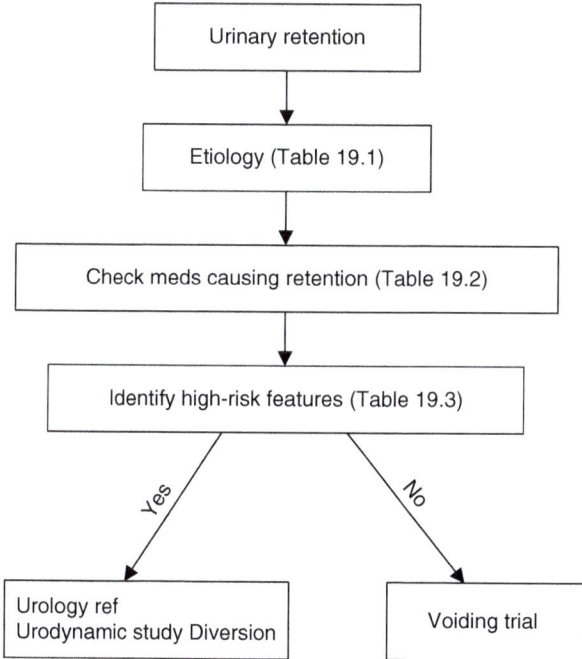

© The Author(s), under exclusive license to Springer Nature Switzerland AG 2025

M. J. Morikawa, *The Inpatient Medicine Handbook*,

https://doi.org/10.1007/978-3-032-08398-2_19

FACTs:

- Acute urinary retention in elderly is related to increased 1 year mortality [1]
- Chronic urinary retention (CUR) = PVR >300 mL documented >2 separate occasions at least 6 months [2]
- 25–60% of DM patient will develop diabetic cystopathy [3]
- CVA more commonly leads to urinary incontinence, but retention more commonly occur in brainstem CVA [3]
- Most common obstructive causes is BPH [4]
- Most common infection is acute prostatitis [3]
- NSAIDs use can cause retention [3]

Table 19.1 Five etiologies

Etiologies	Examples
Obstructive	BPH, uterine prolapse, pelvic mass
ID/Inflammation	Prostatitis, vulvoganinitis, vaginal licken sclerosus, planus, pemphigus
Iatrogenic	Medications, trauma,
Neurologic	CVA, spinal cord lesions, autonomic neuropathy

Selius and Subedi [4]; Serlin et al. [3]

Table 19.2 Meds causing retention

Class	Meds
Antiarrhythmics	Disopyramide, quinidine, procainamide
Anticholinergics	Atropine, oxybutynin, scopolamine, dicyclomine
Antidepressants	Amitriptyline, doxepin, imipramine, nortriptyline
Antihistamines	Diphenhydramine, cyproheptadine, dydroxyzine
Antihypertensives	Hydralazine, nifedipine
Anti PD meds	Amantadine, benztropine, bromocriptine, levodopa
Antipsychotics	Chlorpromazine, haloperidol, thioridazine
Hormonal agents	Estrogen, progesterone, testosterone
Muscle relaxants	Baclofen, cyclobenzaprine, diazepam
Alpha-adrenergic agents	Ephedrine, phenylephrine, pseudoephedrine,
Beta-adrenergic agents	Isoproterenol, metaproterenol, terbutaline
Others	Amphetamine, carbamazepine, NSAIDs

Based on Selius and Subedi [4]; Serlin et al. [3]

Table 19.3 High risk chronic urinary retention

Radiological findings	Laboratory findings	Signs/symptoms
Hydronephrosis hydroureter	Stage 3 CKD Recurrent symptomatic, culture + UTI Culture proven systemic urosepsis	Urinary incontinence with perineal skin changes Urinary incontinence with sacral decubitus ulcers

Stoffel et al. [2]

- High risk patient should be evaluated by urologist including urodynamic studies and consult for permanent drainage

Incontinence

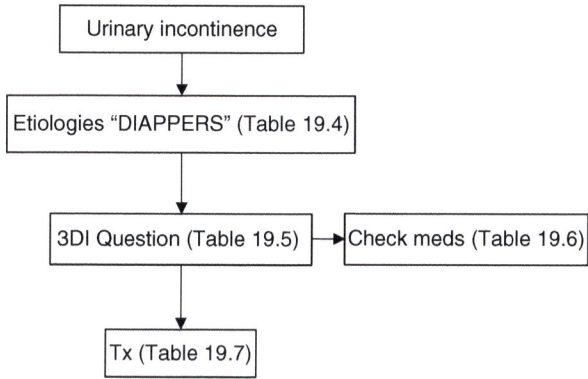

Table 19.4 DDx: DIAPPERS

	Causes
D	Delirium, dementia
I	Infection
A	Atrophic vaginitis, urethritis, alcohol ingestion
P	Psychologic: depression
P	Pharmacologic
E	Endocrine: hypercalcemia, hyperglycemia, excess UO
R	Restricted mobility: physical restraints, fractures
S	Stool impaction

Keilman [5]

Table 19.5 Dx 3QI

"3 questions in 3 months"
1. During the last 3 months, have you leaked urine? Yes or No
2. During the last 3 months, did you leak urine:
(a) Performing physical activity, e.g. coughing, sneezing, lifting or exercise?
(b) Had the urge but couldn't get to the toilet fast enough?
(c) Without activity or urge?
3. During the last 3 months, did you leak urine most often:
(a) Performing some physical activity?
(b) Had urge, but couldn't make it to the toilet?
(c) Without physical activity or urge?
(d) About equally as often with physical activity or urgency?

Brown et al. [6]

- Most often with physical activity: Stress
- Most often with urge to empty bladder: Urge
- Equally physical activity or urge: Mixed
- Without either: other cause

Table 19.6 Meds causing incontinence

Decrease bladder contractility (retention and overflow incontinence)	Meds causing retention + ACEi
Increase detrusor irritability	Alcohol Caffeine Diuretics
Increase urethral sphincter tone	Alpha adrenergic agonist Amphetamines TCA
Decrease urethral sphincter tone	Alpha adrenergic antagonists

Based on Hu and Pierre [7]

Tx for female [8]
- Urge or mixed; Anticholinergic oxybutynin, tolterodine, darifenacin
- Anticholinergic shouldn't be offered to isolated stress symptoms in absence of urge

Table 19.7 Mgmt of Lower urinary tract symptoms (LUTS) in men

Symptoms	Etiology	Mgmt
Urgency, frequency, nocturia	Storage: Overactive bladder	Anticholinergic (antimuscarinics) Solifenacin, tolterodine, oxybutynin $\beta 3$ adrenoceptor agonist mirabegron
Hesitancy, intermittency, slow stream, straining, terminal dribble	Voiding: outflow obstruction (BPH)	α-blocker 5α reductase inhibitor Phosphodiesterase inhibitor
Post-micturition dribble, sensation of incomplete emptying	Post-micturition	Urethral milking to empty bulbar urethra

Rees et al. [9]

Urinary Diversion
Types: three types

Non orthotopic non-continent diversion	Intestinal conduit
Non orthotopic continent diversion	Intestinal pouch (Indiana pouch) Ureterosigmoidostomy
Orthotopic continent diversion	Neobladder (Studer pouch)

Modified from Falagas and Vergidis [10]; Sperling et al. [11]

Recommendations for treatment for different types of diversions

Type of diversion	Organism	Treatment
Noncontinent urinary diversion	G+ mixed skin flora G− Enterobacteriaceae E. faecalis	No Tx unless hx of recurrent pyelonephritis
Continent nonorthotopic diversion	Chronic bacteriuria due to intermittent self-cath	No tx
Orthotopic urinary diversion	E coli and other G− Enterobacteriaceae	No Tx but treat urea-splitting organism e.g. Proteus even if asymptomatic due to potential stone formation

Based on Falagas and Vergidis [10]

References

1. Armitage J, et al. Mortality in men admitted to hospital with acute urinary retention: database analysis. BMJ. 2007. https://doi.org/10.1136/bmj.39377.617269.55.
2. ☺☺Stoffel J, et al. AUA white paper on nonneurogenic chronic urinary retention: consensus definition, treatment algorithm, and outcome end points. J Urol. 2017;198:153–60.
3. ☺☺Serlin D, et al. Urinary retention in adults: evaluation and initial management. Am Fam Physician. 2018;98(8):496–503.
4. Selius B, Subedi R. Urinary retention in adults: diagnosis and initial management. Am Fam Physician. 2008;77:643–50.
5. Keilman L. Urinary incontinence: basic evaluation and management in the primary care office. Prim Care Clin Office Pract. 2005;32:699–722.
6. Brown J, et al. The sensitivity and specificity of a simple test to distinguish between urge and stress urinary incontinence. Ann Intern Med. 2006;144:715–23.
7. Hu J, Pierre E. Urinary incontinence in women: evaluation and management. Am Fam Physician. 2019;100(6):339–48.
8. ☺☺☺Wood L, Anger J. Urinary incontinence in women. BMJ. 2014;349:g4531. https://doi.org/10.1136/bmj.g4531.
9. ☺☺Rees J, et al. The management of lower urinary tract symptoms in men. BMJ. 2014;348:g3861. https://doi.org/10.1136/bmj.g3861.
10. ☺Falagas M, Vergidis P. Urinary tract infections in patients with urinary diversion. Am J Kidney Dis. 2005;46:1030–7.
11. ☺☺☺Sperling C, et al. Urinary diversion: core curriculum 2021. Am J Kidney Dis. 2021;78(2):293–304.

Vascular Medicine

20

PAD

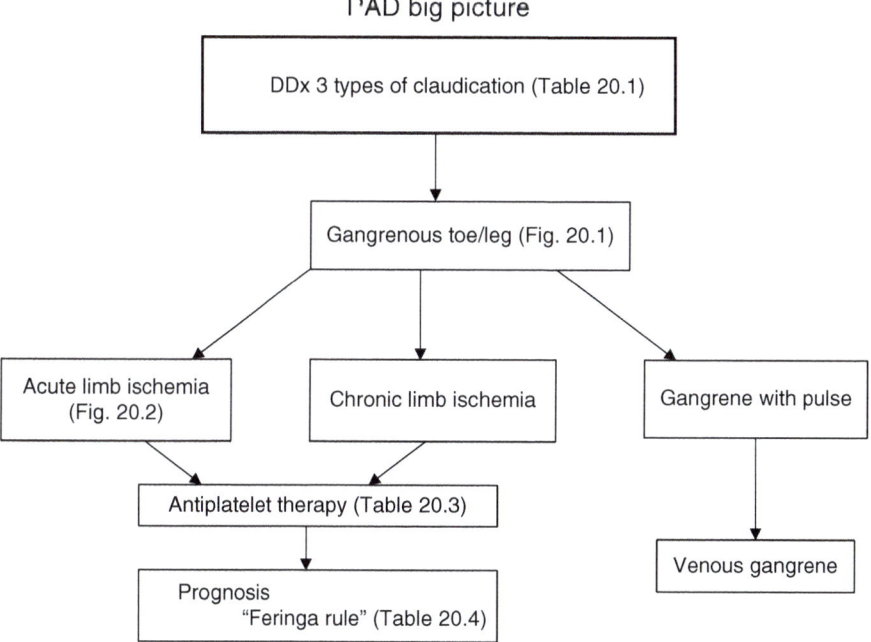

PAD big picture

DDx 3 types of claudication (Table 20.1)

Gangrenous toe/leg (Fig. 20.1)

Acute limb ischemia (Fig. 20.2)

Chronic limb ischemia

Gangrene with pulse

Antiplatelet therapy (Table 20.3)

Prognosis "Feringa rule" (Table 20.4)

Venous gangrene

PAD and ABI

- PAD is defined as ABI ≤0.9 or Toe brachial index ≤0.7 [1]
- ABI >1.3 poorly compressible, calcified arteries [2]
- ABI is predictive for CVD [3]

© The Author(s), under exclusive license to Springer Nature Switzerland AG 2025
M. J. Morikawa, *The Inpatient Medicine Handbook*,
https://doi.org/10.1007/978-3-032-08398-2_20

Table 20.1 Claudication

• Only 15% of PAD patients complained intermittent claudication [1, 4]			
• Different types of claudication [4, 5]			
Characteristics	Intermittent claudication	Venous congestion	Spinal stenosis
Pain character	Cramping, tightness	Bursting pain	Weakness, clumsinessElectric shock-like
Location	Buttock, hip, thigh, calf, foot (muscle groups)	Groin, thighWhole leg	Buttock, hip, thighPoorly localized
Exercise induced discomfort	Yes	After walking	Variable
Relief of discomfort	Rapid relief with rest	Relief sitting or bend forward	Slow relief with leg elevation
Legs affected	Usually one	Usually one	Often both

CLI

- Critical limb ischemia: ABI <0.4 and toe SBP <30 mmHg
- 5–10% of asymptomatic PAD or claudication will progress to CLI in 5 years
- Majority of CLI have infrainguinal disease
- 4 year risk of MI is 10% and CVA is 8% [6–8].

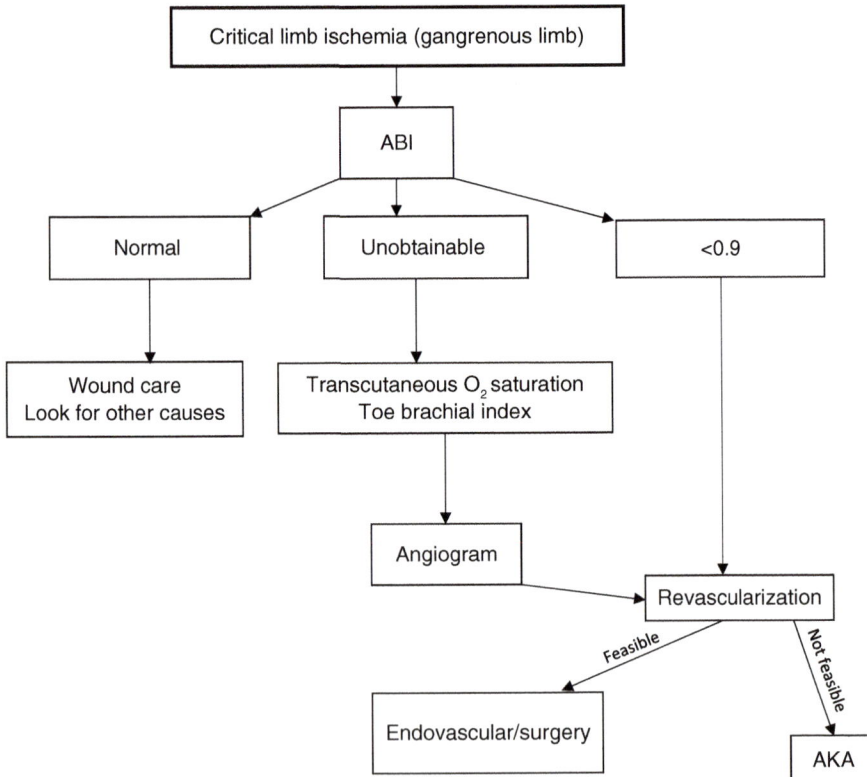

Fig. 20.1 Gangrenous limb

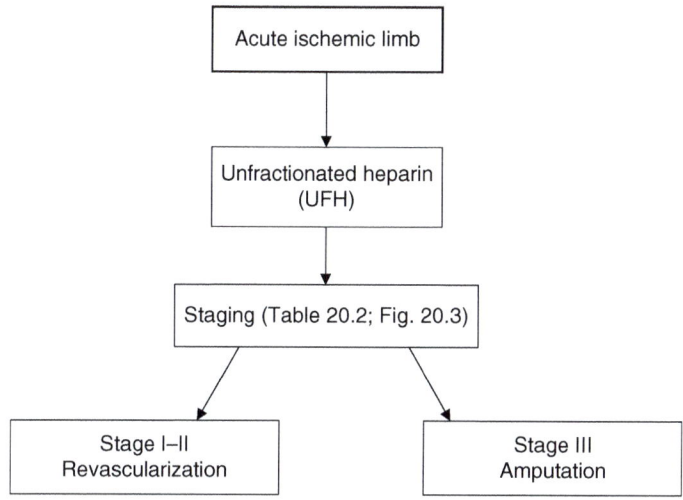

Fig. 20.2   Acute limb ischemia

- Acute limb ischemia has 15–20% mortality in 1-year [6, 9]
- Six Ps: paresthesia, pain, paller, pulselessness, paralysis and poikilothermia
- Reperfusion injury: compartment syndrome

Table 20.2   Staging

	I	II		III
		IIa	IIb	
Description	Viable not threatened	Marginally threatened	Immediately threatenedSalvageable with immediate intervention	Irreversibly damagedMajor tissue loss
Sensory loss	–	Only toe or none	More than toe pain at rest	Profound, anesthetic
Muscle weakness	–	–	++	Paralysis
Arterial doppler	+	±	–	–
Venous doppler	+	+	+	–

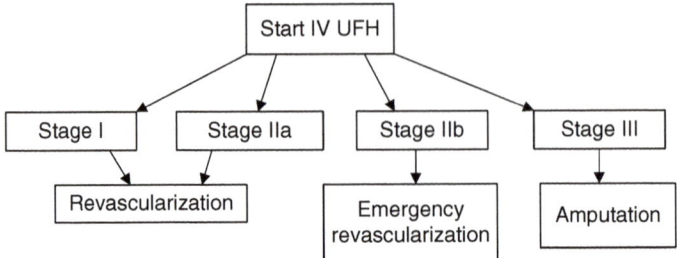

Fig. 20.3 Mgmt

Anatomical correlation and Level of arterial involvement [2]
Three arteries and six agniosomes in leg [8]

SMK/HTN—aortoiliac A
DM—infrapopliteal
Vasculitis—micro or terminal A

Buttock/hip pain—aortoiliac A
Thigh—iliofemoral
Upper 2/3 calf—superficial femoral
Lower 1/3 calf—popliteal
Foot—tibial/peroneal A

Table 20.3 Antithrombotic mgmt of PAD

Asymptomatic	Symptomatic		Revascularization	
	All patients	Recent ACS	Surgical	Endovascular
Consider ASA	ASA or clopidogrel or ASA + rivaroxaban	DAPT		DAPT × 1–6 months
			ASA or clopidogrel or ASA + Rivaroxaban	

Hussain [10]

High Limb Risk

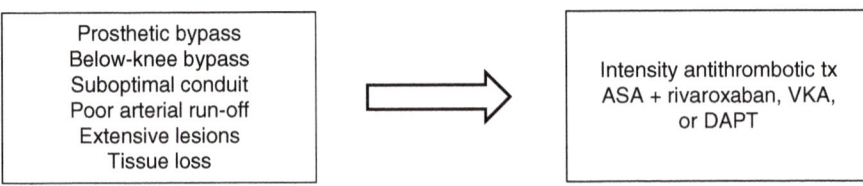

Prosthetic bypass
Below-knee bypass
Suboptimal conduit
Poor arterial run-off
Extensive lesions
Tissue loss

Intensity antithrombotic tx
ASA + rivaroxaban, VKA,
or DAPT

Prognosis

Table 20.4 Feringa rule

• 1-year and 5-year mortality prediction		
Risk factors:		
	1-year mortality risk score	5-year mortality risk score
Age >65	+15	+7
Cr >2.0 or HD	+15	+15
Total chol >212.4 mg/dL	+13	+5
Hx of CHF	+9	+8
ABI <0.6	+8	+7
Q wave	+7	+3
DM	+6	+4
ß blocker use	−6	−4
ASA use	−8	−7
Statins	−18	−6
Hx of CVA	–	+7
ST change	–	+5

Outcome			
	Score	1-year mortality	5-year mortality
Low	< 1 (1-year) <1 (5-year)	0.6	6.9
Low-intermediate	1–13 (1-year) 1–7 (5-year)	2.7	16.2
High-intermediate	14–22 (1-year) 8–14 (5-year)	7.4	23.2
High	22 < (1-year) 14 < (5-year)	17.8	52.5

Feringa et al. [11]

Carotid Artery (Fig. 20.4)

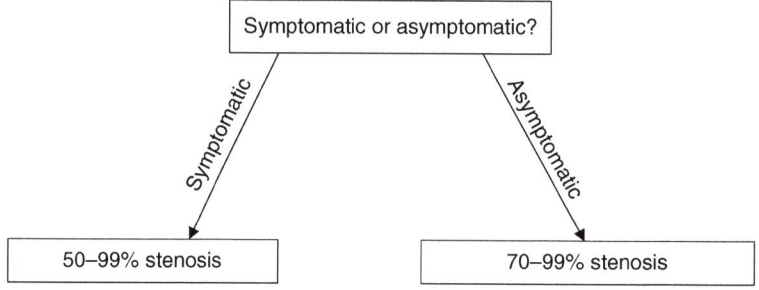

Fig. 20.4 Indication for intervention

- Symptomatic patients 50–99% stenosis or asymptomatic pt 70–99% should be stented (CAS) [12]
- Symptomatic patients with >70% stenosis should get intervention <2 weeks [13] (Fig. 20.5)

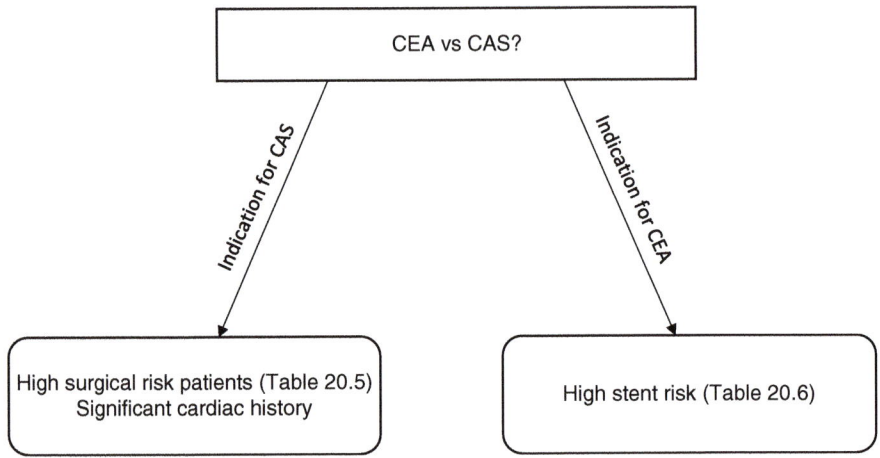

Fig. 20.5   CEA vs CAS

Table 20.5   Indication for carotid artery stent (CAS)

=Those with high-risk for CEA get CAS	
Clinical	Anatomic
CHF NYHA class III/IV	Surgically inaccessible lesion
Unstable angina	Ipsilateral neck irradiation
CAD with LM or ≥2 vessels ≥70% stenosis	Spinal immobility of the neck
Recent MI (≤30 days)	Contralateral carotid occlusion
Planned open heart surgery (≤30 days)	Contralateral laryngeal palsy
LVEF ≤30%	Tracheostoma
Severe pulmonary disease	Prior ipsilateral CEA or neck surgery
Severe renal disease	

- Significant cardiac issues

Table 20.6   Indication for carotid endarterectomy (CEA)

=high-risk for CAS	
Clinical	Anatomic
Elderly (>75)	High-grade aortic arch atheroma
Bleeding disorder	Type II/III aortic arch
Severe AS	Stenosis at origin of great vessels
Severe renal disease	≥2 acute bends (90°)
Decreased cerebral reserve	Circumferential lesion calcification
Dementia	Lesion-related thrombus
	Tandem lesions
	Lack of femoral access
	Unable to use EPD (embolic protection device)

• Elderly >75, tortuous, calcified artery

    White et al. [12]; Meschia et al. [14]

AORTA
AAA (Fig. 20.6; Tables 20.7 and 20.8)

Diameter >5.5 cm should be referred to vascular surgeon

Metcalfe et al. [15]

Fig. 20.6   Risk of rupture by size: NON-LINEAR!

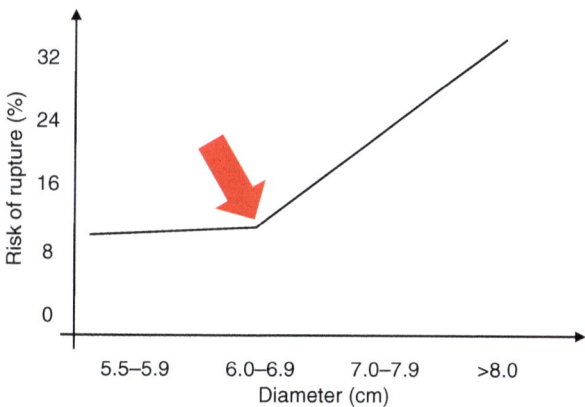

Table 20.7   Annual rupture rate

5.5–5.9 cm	6.0–6.9 cm (6.5–6.9 cm)	≥7.0 cm
9.4%	10.2% (19.1%)	32.5%

Metcalfe et al. [15]; Lederle et al. [16]

Table 20.8 Surveillance intervals

3.0–3.9 cm	4.0–4.9 cm	≥5.0 cm
Q3 year	Yearly	Q6 month

Schanzer and Oderich [17]; The RESCAN Collaborators [18]; Chaikof et al. [19]

AAS (Acute Aortic Syndrome)
Chest pain and 'triple rule out by CTPA' (Fig. 20.7)

Table 20.9 *AAS*

EKG change	Troponin	D-dimer	Hypoxia	
–	±	+	+	PE
+	+	–	–	ACS
–	–	+	–	AAS

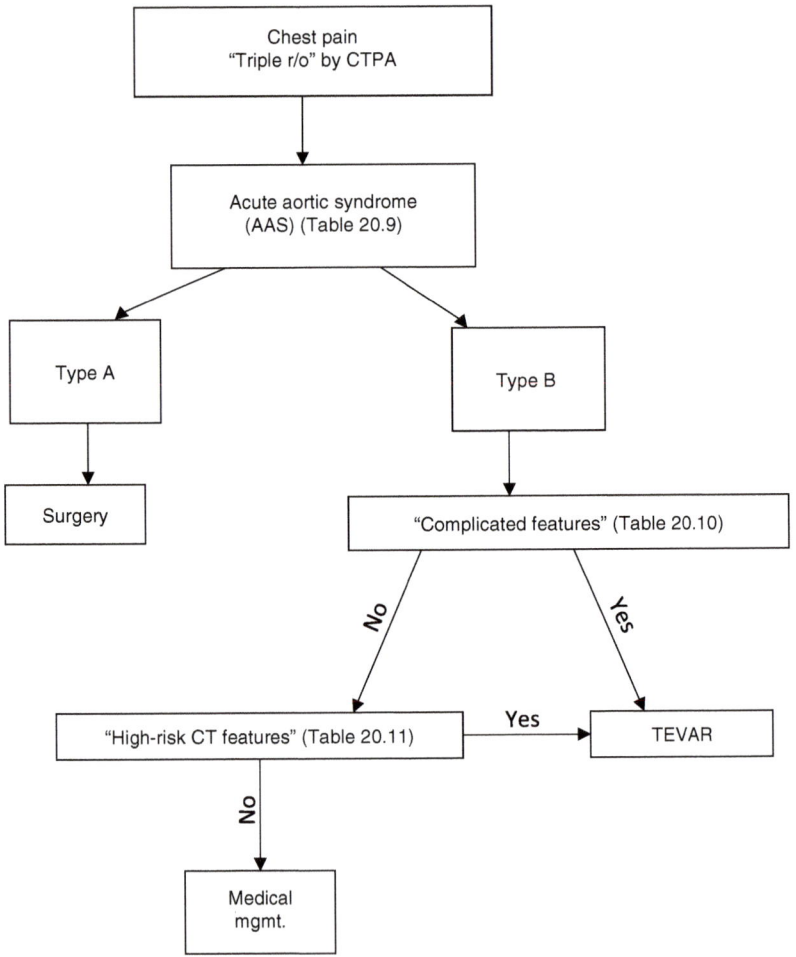

Fig. 20.7 AAS algorithm

Acute aortic syndrome (AAS) [20] (classification [21, 22])

1. Aortic dissection (AD)
2. Intramural hematoma (IMH)
3. Penetrating aortic ulcer (PAU) (Fig. 20.8)

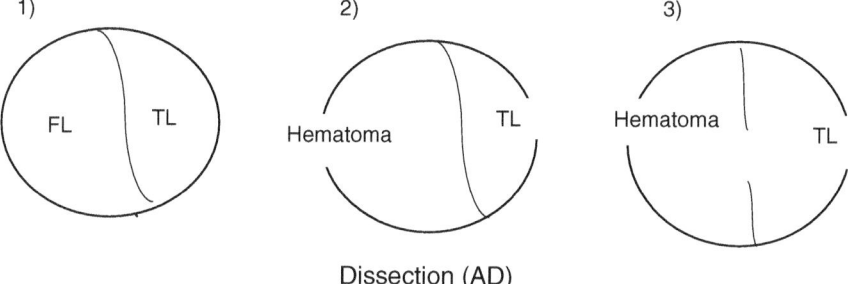

Dissection (AD)

Fig. 20.8 *AAS*

Classification (DeBakey, Stanford) (Fig. 20.9)

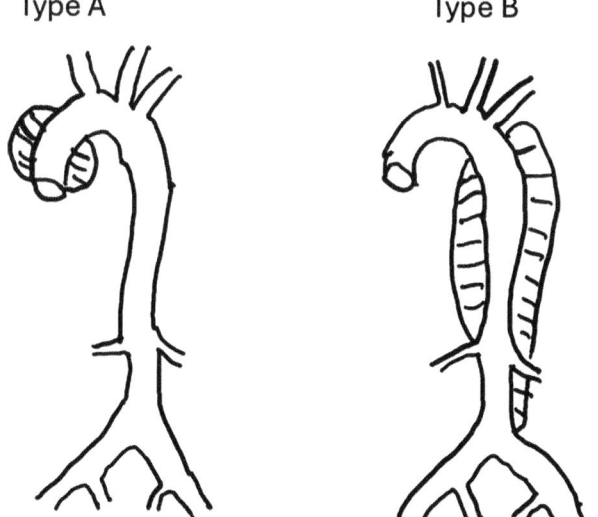

Fig. 20.9   Stanford Type A and B [20, 21]

Biomarker

- Negative D-dimer can rule out dissection [23]

Strategy [20, 23, 24]

- IV beta-blocker: Labetalol [24]
  Stanford type A—surgery
  Stanford type B—TEVAR/medical mgmt

Table 20.10 Complicated type B features

Aortic rupture
End-organ ischemia
Continuing pain and HTN despite medical tx
Early false lumen expansion
Large single entry of entry tear

Nienaber and Clough [23]

Table 20.11 "High risk feature of CT findings" for late aortic complication

Primary entry tear diameter >10 mm
Initial total aortic diameter ≥40 mm
False lumen diameter ≥22 mm
Patent false lumen (vs. fully thrombosed)
Partially thrombosed false lumen

Tadros et al. [24]

Splanchnic Artery Aneurysm

- More common than AAA.
- Splenic artery aneurysm is the most common
- Distribution Fig. 20.6
- Intervention if >2 cm in diameter, pregnant or sign of growth (Table 20.12)

Table 20.12 Distribution/frequency

Location	Frequency (%)
Splenic A	60
Proper hepatic A	20
SMA	5.5
Celiac A	4
Gastric/Gastroepiploic A	4
Other location	<3

Pasha et al. [25]

Acute Mesenteric Ischemia (AMI)

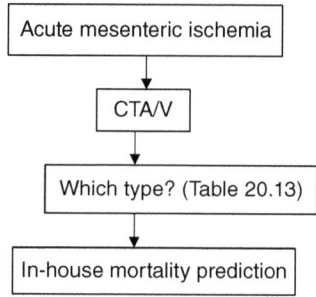

Arterial—endovascular vs surgery
Venous—anticoagulation
NOMI—treat underlying causes (Table 20.14)

Table 20.13 Four types of AMI

Type	Incidence	Symptoms	Presentation	RFs	Mortality
Arterial embolism (AE)	34%	Acute onset N/V Diarrhea Hematochezia	Pain out of proportion Peritonitis Hypotension Tachycardia	Af, hxo MI, CHF, Prior AE	70%
Arterial thrombosis (AT)	34%	Progressively worse pain Food fear Weight loss Postprandial pain	N/V diarrhea Cramping, periumblical pain	Chronic symptoms, hx of CAD, PAD SMK	66%
Mesenteric Venous thrombosis (MVT)	15%	Insidious onset Vague abdominal pain	Vague tenderness GI bleeding	Prior VTE Recent abdominal surgery Known hypercoagulable state	44%
Nonocclusive mesenteric ischemia (NOMI)	18%	Critically ill patient with abdominal pin Hypotension Altered mental status	Tenderness Distension Feeding intolerance	Recent cardiac surgery ESRD Low EF Digitalis vasopressors	70%

Russell et al. [27]; Carver et al. [28]; Clair and Beach [29]

Table 20.14 In-house mortality prediction

Variable		Score	
Age			
≥70		1	
EKG			
Af 60–90/min		2	
Any other abnormal rhythm or >4/min ectopies or Q was and ST/T change		4	
Shock index			
≥0.7 (HR/SBP)		2	
Score	≤2	3–4	5 ≤
Mortality	19%	37%	91%

Haga et al. [26]

Vein

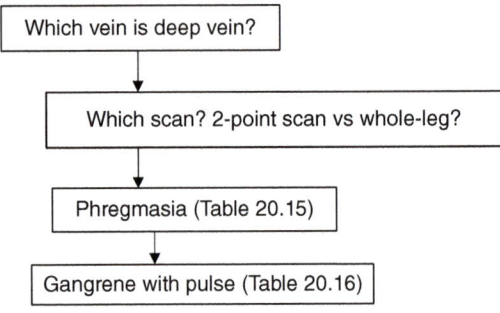

Deep Vein

Upper extremity

- UE: IJ, Subclavian, Brachiocephalic, Axillary, Brachial (External jugular, Cephalic or Basilic are NOT) [30]
- PE, recurrence at 12 months is less common in the UE than in the LE [31]

Lower extremity [32]

- 20% of patients with PE have proximal DVT [33]
- Deep vein: common femoral, superficial femoral, popliteal, peroneal and posterior tibial [34]

Different methods of scanning of LE [34]

- 2-point scan + D-dimer and whole-leg scan doesn't make difference in outcome [35, 36]

Table 20.15 Phregmasia

Phlegmasia alba dolens	White leg	Extensive DVT (No tissue ischemia since superficial collateral vessels preserved)	
Phlegmasia cerula dolens	Blue leg	Complete obstruction of both superficial and deep venous return (tissue ischemia +)	Resultant severe venous congestion leads to increased pressure on small arterioles and to tissue ischemia Cyanotic or dusky appearance, gangrene

Gillenwater et al. [37]; Gibson et al. [38]

Gangrene with pulse

- Thrombosis involving microcirculation causes limb necrosis without thrombo-embolism of arteries
- There are two forms of microthrombosis-associated limb ischemia and gangrene: venous limb gangrene and peripheral symmetric gangrene (Table 20.16).
- These two forms are cutaneous manifestation of underlying DIC.
- Microthrombosis occurs in the same limb with acute large vein thrombosis resulting in distal extremity (acral) ischemic necrosis.

Table 20.16 Ischemic limb with pulse

	Venous limb gangrene	Symmetric peripheral gangrene
Etiology	HITT, metastatic cancer, antiphospholipid syndrome	Septic shock, cardiogenic shock
DVT	+	–
location	One limb	Usually symmetrical 2 or 4 limbs

Warkentin [39]

Varicose vein

- Symptoms of varicose veins increase with age [40]
- Skin changes are (1) eczema; (2) hemosiderin deposition; (3) atrophie blanche or hypopigmentation; and (4) lipodermatosclerosis with upside-down champagne bottle appearance [41]
- Corona phlebectatica is an early sign of advanced venous disease [42]

References

1. ☺Campia U, et al. Peripheral artery disease: past, present, and future. Am J Med. 2019;132:1133–41.
2. Arain F, Cooper L. Peripheral arterial disaese: diagnosis and management. Mayo Clin Proc. 2008;83:944–50.
3. Mehler P, et al. Intensive blood pressure control reduces the risk of cardiovascular events in patients with peripheral arterial disease and type 2 diabetes. Circulation. 2003;107:753–6.
4. ☺☺☺White C. Intermittent claudication. N Engl J Med. 2007;356:1241–50.
5. Burns P, et al. Management of peripheral arterial disease in primary care. BMJ. 2003;326:584–8.
6. ☺Norgren L, et al. Inter-society consensus for the management of peripheral arterial disease (TASC II). J Vasc Surg. 2007;45 Suppl S(1):S5A–67A.
7. ☺☺Farber A. Chronic limb-threatening ischemia. N Engl J Med. 2018;379:171–80.
8. Shishehbor M, et al. Critical limb ischemia. J Am Coll Cardiol. 2016;68:2002–15.
9. ☺☺☺Creager M, et al. Acute limb ischemia. N Engl J Med. 2012;366:2198–206.
10. ☺☺☺Hussain M, et al. Antithrombotic therapy for peripheral artery disease. Recent advances. J Am Coll Cardiol. 2018;71:2450–67.
11. Feringa H, et al. A prognostic risk index for long-term mortality in patients with peripheral arterial disease. Arch Intern Med. 2007;167(22):2482–9.
12. ☺☺☺White C, et al. Carotid artery stenting. J Am Coll Cardiol. 2022;80:155–70.
13. ☺Grotta J. Carotid stenosis. N Engl J Med. 2013;369:1143–50.
14. ☺☺Meschia J, et al. Evaluation and management of atherosclerotic carotid stenosis. Mayo Clin Proc. 2017;92(7):1144–57.
15. Metcalfe D, et al. The management of abdominal aortic aneurysms. BMJ. 2011;342:d1384. https://doi.org/10.1136/bmj.d1384.
16. Lederle F, et al. Rupture rate of large abdominal aortic aneurysms in patients refusing or unfit for elective repair. JAMA. 2002;287:2968–72.
17. ☺☺☺Schanzer A, Oderich G. Management of abdominal aortic aneurysm. N Engl J Med. 2021;385:1690–8.
18. The RESCAN Collaborators. Surveillance intervals for small abdominal aortic aneurysms. A meta-analysis. JAMA. 2013;309(8):806–13.
19. ☺☺Chaikof E, et al. SVS practice guidelines for the care of patients with an abdominal aortic aneurysm: executive summary. J Vasc Surg. 2009;50(4):880–96.
20. Mussa F, et al. Acute aortic dissection and intramural hematoma. A systematic review. JAMA. 2016;316(7):754–63.
21. Thrumurthy S, et al. The diagnosis and management of aortic dissection. BMJ. 2012;344:d8290.
22. ☺☺☺Vilacosta I, et al. Acute aortic syndrome revisited. J Am Coll Cardiol. 2021;78:2106–25.
23. Nienaber C, Clough R. Management of acute aortic dissection. Lancet. 2015;385:800–11.
24. ☺☺Tadros R, et al. Optimal treatment of uncomplicated Type B aortic dissection. J Am Coll Cardiol. 2019;74:1494–504.
25. ☺Pasha S, et al. Splanchnic artery aneurysms. Mayo Clin Proc. 2007;82:472–9.
26. Haga Y, et al. New prediction rule for mortality in acute mesenteric ischemia. Digestion. 2009;80:104–11.
27. Russell C, et al. Mesenteric venous thrombosis. Circulation. 2015;131:1599–603.
28. ☺☺Carver T, et al. Mesenteric ischemia. Crit Care Clin. 2016;32:155–71.
29. Clair D, Beach J. Mesenteric ischemia. N Engl J Med. 2016;374:959–68.
30. Mai C, Hunt D. Upper-extremity deep venous thrombosis: a review. Am J Med. 2011;124:402–7.
31. ☺Kucher N. Deep-vein thrombosis of the upper extremities. N Engl J Med. 2011;364:861–9.
32. van den Boezem P, et al. The management of superficial venous incompetence. BMJ. 2011;343:d4489. https://doi.org/10.1136/bmj.d4489.
33. ☺☺Konstantinides S. Acute pulmonary embolism. N Engl J Med. 2008;359:2804–13.
34. Needleman L, et al. Ultrasound for lower extremity deep venous thrombosis. Circulation. 2018;137:1505–15.

35. ☺ ☺ Bernardi E, et al. Serial 2-point ultrasonography plus D-dimer vs whole-leg color-coded doppler ultrasonography for diagnosing suspected symptomatic deep vein thrombosis. A randomized controlled trial. JAMA. 2008;300:1653–9.
36. Sevestre M, et al. Outcomes for inpatients with normal findings on whole-leg ultrasonography: a prospective study. Am J Med. 2010;123:158–65.
37. Gillenwater J, et al. Phlegmasia cerulea dolens. Circulation. 1962;25:39–42.
38. Gibson C, et al. Out of the blue. N Engl J Med. 2014;370:1742–8.
39. ☺ ☺ ☺ Warkentin T. Ischemic limb gangrene with pulses. N Engl J Med. 2015;373:642–55.
40. Bradbury A, et al. What are the symptoms of varicose veins? Edinburgh vein study cross sectional population survey. BMJ. 1999;318:353–6.
41. Atkins E, et al. Varicose veins in primary care. BMJ. 2020;370:m2509. https://doi.org/10.1136/bmj.m2509.
42. Raetz J, et al. Varicose veins: diagnosis and treatment. Am Fam Physician. 2019;99(11):682–8.

Transplant Patient 21

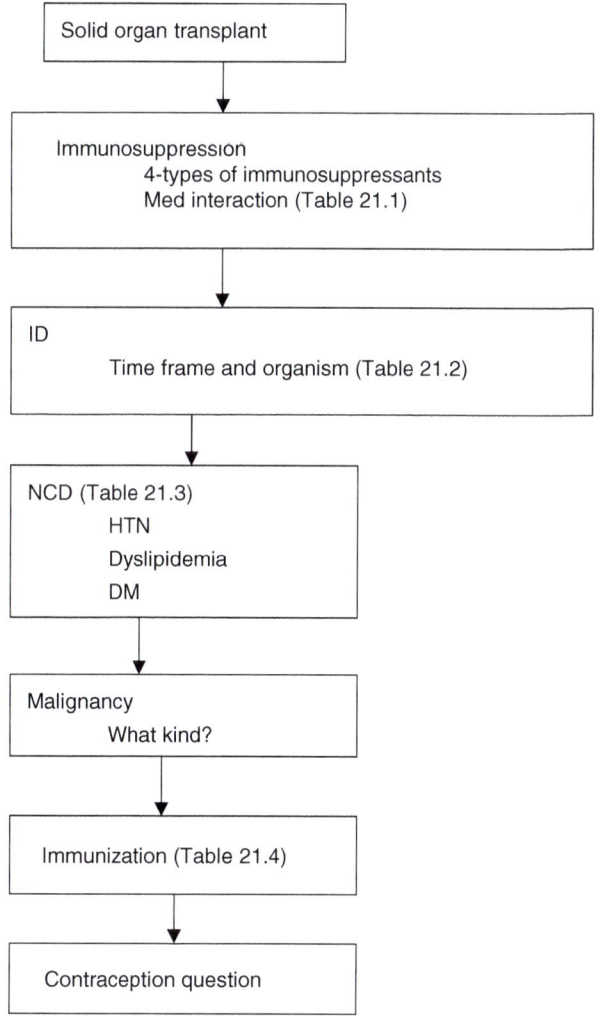

- Liver transplant mortality lowest in PBS, highest in cancer [1]
- For etiology of mortality at 1 year post liver transplant, refer to [2]

Immunosuppression

Table 21.1 Medication interaction with CIN

Important interactions with tacrolimus, ciclosporin, or rapamycin	
Inhibit P450 and ↑ blood level	Erythromycin, clarithromycin, clotrimazole, fluconazole, ketoconazole
	Rifampin
	Grapefruit juice
	Diltiazem, verapamil, nicardipine
	Metoclopramide
	Ranitidine
Induce P450 and ↓ blood level	Warfarin
	Phenytoin, phenobarbital, carbamazepine
	INH, Nafcillin

Based on Hasley and Arnold [3]; Hirschfield et al. [1]

- Three signals of immune activation, Kant et al. [4] and Lien [5]
- Immunosuppresants and CVD risk, [6]

ID
Fischer [7]

Fishman [8]: donor related; recipient driven; nosocomial; community

O'Shea and Humar [9]

Foster and Fosger [10]

Guenette and Husain [11]

Timsit et al. [12]

Table 21.2 Time frame and pathogens

<1 month	1–6 month	6 month <
Nosocomial	Opportunistic	Community
MRSA	CMV, BK, EBV, HSV	CMV, JC
VRE	CDI, VZV, crypto, legionella	
Aspergillosis	HSV	

NCD

Table 21.3 Mgmt of NCD

HTN	Dyslipidemia	DM
CIN increases risk of HTN 60–70% of SOT [3] Cyclosporine >> taclorimus for HTN [13] CCB >>> ACEI/ARB [13] Hydropyridine CCB increases level of CIN [14] BP goal 130/80 < [14, 15]	60–90% prevalence Pravastatin [3, 6] 45–49% develop dyslipidemia and goal is with CAD <100, other <130 [2]	Prevalence of DM is 53% in liver transplant [3] Taclorimus has 70% higher incidence of DM in post transplant [6] CVA is the leading cause of mortality in SOT [14]

Malignancy
- Skin cancers are the most common after liver transplant, followed by PTLD [2]
- PTLD has six subclasses [16]
- Post transplant erythrocytosis in renal transplant if Ht >51% [5]
- HVGD [17]

Immunization
- Live vaccine is contraindicated [3, 18]

Table 21.4 Immunization

Pneumococcus	Unvaccinated before transplant A dose of PCV13 followed 2 months later 1 dose of PPV23	Vaccinated before transplant 1 dose of PPV23 at least 5 years after the first dose of PPV23
Influenza	Tetravalent inactivated vaccine Q year	
HAV	Unvaccinated before transplant: 2 doses 6–12 months apart	
HBV	Unvaccinated before transplant: 3 doses, at 0, 1, 6 months	
HPV	Female 9–45 years unvaccinated: 3 doses at 0, 2, and 6 months	
Tdap	Q 10 years	

Based on Toniutto et al. [18]

Contraception
- Progesterone only recommended, estrogen should be avoided since it may raise BP and may increase the blood levels of CNI [5, 14].

References

1. Hirschfield G, et al. Adult liver transplantation: what non-specialists need to know. BMJ. 2009;338:1321–7.
2. ☺☺Singh S, Watt K. Long-term medical management of the liver transplant recipient: what the primary care physician needs to know. Mayo Clin Proc. 2012;87(8):779–90.
3. ☺☺☺Hasley P, Arnold R. Primary care of the transplant patient. Am J Med. 2010;123:205–12.
4. Kant S, et al. Management of hospitalized kidney transplant recipient for hospitalists and internists. Am J Med. 2022;135:950–7.
5. Lien Y. Top 10 things primary care physicians should know about maintenance immunosuppression for transplant recipients. Am J Med. 2016;129:568–72.
6. Sen A, et al. Complications of solid organ transplantation. Cardiovascular, neurologic, renal and gastrointestinal. Crit Care Clin. 2019;35:169–86.
7. ☺Fischer S. Infections complicating solid organ transplantation. Surg Clin North Am. 2006;86:1127–45.
8. ☺☺☺Fishman J. Infection in solid-organ transplant recipients. N Engl J Med. 2007;357:2601–14.
9. O'Shea D, Humar A. Life-threatening infection in transplant recipients. Crit Care Clin. 2013;29:953–73.
10. Foster J, Foster K. Care of the renal transplant patient. Prim Care Clin Office Pract. 2020;47:703–12.
11. Guenette A, Husain S. Infectious complications following solid organ transplantation. Crit Care Clin. 2019;35:151–68.
12. Timsit J, et al. Diagnostic and therapeutic approach to infectious diseases in solid organ transplant recipients. Intensive Care Med. 2019;45:573–91.
13. Mangray M, Vella J. Hypertension after kidney transplant. Am J Kidney Dis. 2011;57(2):331–41.
14. Cimino F, Snyder K. Primary care of the solid organ transplant recipient. AFP. 2016;93(3):203–10.
15. Nieto T, et al. Renal transplantation in adults. BMJ. 2016;355:i6158. https://doi.org/10.1136/bmj.i6158.
16. ☺Dierickx D, Habermann T. Post-transplant lymphoproliferative disorders in adults. N Engl J Med. 2018;378:549–62.
17. Zeiser R, Blazar B. Acute graft-versus-host disease- biologic process, prevention, and therapy. N Engl J Med. 2017;377:2167–79.
18. Toniutto P, et al. An essential guide for managing post-liver transplant patients: what primary care physicians should know. Am J Med. 2022;135:157–66.

Part III

Essential Topics

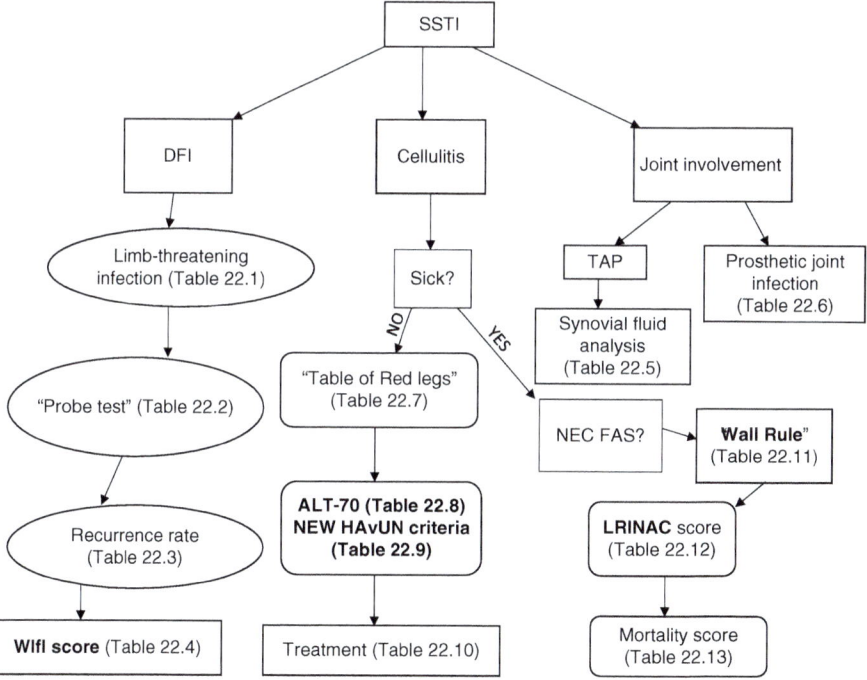

Anatomy of skin and depth of infection:
Impetigo
Ecthyma
Erisipela
Cellulitis
Fasciitis

DFI/Osteo

Table 22.1 "Limb-threatening infection" requiring hospitalization

Limb-threatening infection
Full-thickness ulcer >2 cm of cellulitis
With/without lymphangitis
Bone/joint involvement
Systemic toxicity
Serious ischemia
Unreliable/poor family support

Caputo et al. [1]

Table 22.2 Clinical findings increase likelihood of osteomyelitis

Clinical findings	Positive likelihood ratio
ESR >70 mm/h	11
Ulcer >2 cm	7.2
Positive probe test	6.4

Butalia et al. [2]

- DM-related amputation has >70% of mortality in 5 years and 74% in 2 years if pt. is on RRT [3]

Table 22.3 Recurrence rate of DFI

Post-healing follow up	Recurrence rate
<1 year	40%
3 year	60%
5 year	65%

Classification: WIfI
Wound
Ischemia
Foot Infection

Wound

Table 22.4 WIfI classification and 1 year risk of amputation

Grade	Ulcer	Gangrene
0	None	None
1	Small, shallow	None
2	Deeper ulcer with exposed bone, joint or tendon	limited to digits
3	Extensive, deep ulcer involving forefoot or midfoot	Extensive gangrene involves forefoot and/or midfoot

Ischemia

Grade	ABI	Ankle systolic pressure (mmHg)	Toe pressure (mmHg)
0	≥0.8	>100	≥60
1	0.6–0.79	70–100	40–59
2	0.4–0.59	50–70	30–39
3	≤0.39	<50	<30

Foot Infection

Grade	Clinical presentation
0	No infection
1	≥2 of the following
	Local swelling/induratin
	0.5 cm < Erythema ≤2 cm around the ulcer
	Local tenderness or pain
	Local warmth
	Purulent discharge
2	Erythema >2 cm
	Involving deeper than skin and subcutaneous structure
	No SIRS
3	≥2 SIRS criteria
	Temp >38 or < 36
	HR > 90
	RR > 20 or $PaCO_2 < 32$
	WBC > 12,000 or < 4000

Clinical Stage and Risk of Amputation

Stage	Risk	W	I	fI
1	Very low	0	0	0,1
		0	1	0
		1	0	0,1
		1	1	0
2	Low	0	0	2
		0	1	1
		0	2	0,1
		0	3	0
		1	0	2
		1	1	1
		1	2	0
		2	0	0,1
3	Moderate	0	0	3
		0	2	1,2
		0	3	1,2
		1	0	3
		1	1	2
		1	2	1
		1	3	0,1
		2	0	2
		2	1	0,1
		2	2	0
		3	0	0,1
4	High	0	1,2,3	3
		1	1	3
		1	2,3	2,3
		2	0	3
		2	1	2,3
		2	2	1,2,3
		2	3	0,1,2,3
		3	0	2,3
		3	1,2,3	0,1,2,3

Armstrong et al. [18]; Mills [19]; van Rijen Eur J Vasc Endovasc Surg [20]

Prognosis (1-year amputation rate) based on clinical stage

WIfI stage	I	II	III	IV
Amputation rate	0	8%	11%	38%

van Reijen Eur J Vasc Endovasc Surg (2019)

Septic Joint and Surgical Implants

Table 22.5 Synovial fluid analysis

WBC < 2000	WBC 50,000<	WBC 100,000<
OA	Septic arthritis strongly susp	Definitively septic arthritis

Earwood et al. [4]

Either of the two:

1. ×2 positive cultures of the same organism
2. sinus tract communicating to the joint or visualization of the prosthesis

If not above, use following scoring 'PREOPERATIVE SCORE'.

Table 22.6 Diagnostic for prosthetic joint infection (PJI)

Variable	Point
Serum	2
↑ CRP (>1 mg/dL) or D-dimer (>860 ng/mL)	1
↑ ESR (> 30 mm/h)	
Synovial	3
↑ synovial WBC (>3000 cells/µL) or leukocyte esterase (++)	3
+ alpha-defensin	2
↑ synovial PMN (%) (>80%)	1
↑ synovial CRP (>6.9 mg/L)	

Decision

Scores	Decision
≥6	Infected
2–5	inconclusive (proceed with operative score below)
0–1	Not infected

Intraoeprative Score (+ Preoperative Scores)

Variable	Score
+ histology	3
+ purulence	3
Single positive culture	2

Decision

Scores	Decision
≥ 6	Infected
4–5	inconclusive (consider further molecular testing such as next-generation sequencing)
≤3	Not infected

Parvizi et al. [5]

Cellulitis
- 'red legs' are misdiagnosed as cellulitis in 28–30% of cases [6]
- DDx [6–8]

Table 22.7 "Table of red legs (arms)"

	Unilateral	Bilateral
Infectious	Necrotizing infection Deeper tissue infection Septic arthropathy Unusual infection (erythema migrans, hepes virus)	Bilateral cellulitis Infected ulcers
Non-infectious	Drug eruption Contact dermatitis Vascular causes (DVT, superficial phlebitis, lymphedema, erythromelalgia, calciphylaxis, acrocyanosis, chilblain, Statis dermatitis, lipodermatosclerosis, Crystal arthropathy Carcinoma erysipeloides Paget disease Insect bite	Drug eruption Contact dermatitis Vascular (erythromelagia) Systemic inflammatory disease Sweet's syndrome Well's syndrome

- CRP is better indicator than WBC but not specific [8, 9]
- Score > 4 have >82% PLR

Table 22.8 ALT 70 score

Variable	Point
Asymmetric	3
Age ≥ 70	2
Leukocytosis ≥10	1
Tachycardia ≥90	1

Points and Decision

Points	Decision
0–2	Cellulitis unlikely
3–4	Indeterminant
5–7	Treat as cellulitis

Raff et al. [10]

New onset
Erythema
Warmth
Hx of associated trauma
Ache
Unilaterality
Number of WBC

Table 22.9 NEW HAvUN score

Variable	Point
Acute onset ≤3 day	1
Erythema: pink to light red erythema resulting from microvascular dilation	1
Pyrexia >100.4 °F	1
Hx of associated trauma, mechanical, surgical, bite, burn	1
Ache: tenderness to light touch	1
Unilaterality: single lower extremity	1
Leukocytosis: WBC > 10.0	1

- Score ≥ 4 had sensitivity 100%, specificity 95% for cellulitis [11]

Treatment
- Nonpurulent cellulitis should be treated with antistreptococcal Abx.
- Purulent drainage is most commonly by Staph aureus and empirical coverage for CAMRSA is recommended and empiric therapy for Strep is unnecessary [12]
- Treatment strategy in both purulent or nonpurulent starts with clinical stratification, mild, moderate and severe with SIRS criteria [8]

Table 22.10 Treatment

	Mild	Moderate		Severe
	No systemic signs of infection (0 SIRS)	SIRS≥1		≥2 SIRS + hypotension or immunocompromise or rapid progression
		1 SIRS	≥2 SIRS	
Non-purulent	Oral Abx Cephalexin, dicloxacillin, pen VK	Oral Abx Cephalexin, dicloxacillin, pen VK Oral Abx	IV Abx Cefazolin, CTX, Pen G	IV Abx broad coverage Vanc/zosyn If suspect MRSA IV vanc If prob. strep+MSSA IV cefazolin, CTX
Purulent	Oral Abx	Oral Abx	IV Abx	IV Abx Bread coverage Vanc, linezolid, daptomycin
MSSA	Cephalexin, dicloxacillin,	Cephalexin dicloxacillin	Oxacillin, nafcillin, cefazolin	IV oxacillin, nafcillin, cefazolin or CTX
MRSA	TMX-SFZ doxy	TMX-SF doxy	Vanc, linezolid	Vanc.linezolid, dapto

Necrotizing fasciitis

Table 22.11 Wall criteria

Na > 134 and WBC < 15.5 had 99% NPV.

Wall et al. [13]

- Type I: polymicrobial, type II: monomicrobial [14]
- LRINEC (Laboratory risk indicator for necrotizing fasciitis) score [15, 16]

Table 22.12 LRINEC score

Variable	Point
CRP (mg/dL)	
<15	0
>15	4
WBC	
<15	0
15–25	1
>25	2
Hb(g/dL)	
>13.5	0
11–13.5	1
<11	2
Sodium (mmol/L)	
≥135	0
<135	2
Creatinine (mg/dL)	
≤1.6	0
>1.6	2
Glucose (mg/dL)	
≤180	0
>180	1

Risk category	LRINEC points	Probability
Low	≤5	<50%
Intermediate	6–7	50–75%
High	≥8	≥75%

Table 22.13 Outcome predictor for necrotizing fasciitis

Variable	Point
HR > 110	1
Temperature < 36 °C	1
Serum creatinine >1.5 mg/dL	1
WBC > 40,000 μL	3
Hematocrit >50%	3
Age > 50	3

Outcome

Points	Mortality (%)
0–2	6
3–5	24
≥6	88

Hussein and Anaya [17]

References

1. Caputo G, et al. Assessment and management of foot disease in patients with diabetes. N Engl J Med. 1994;331:854–60.
2. ☺Butalia S, et al. Does this patient with diabetes have osteomyelitis of the lower extremity? JAMA. 2008;299:806–13.
3. ☺☺☺Armstrong D, et al. Diabetic foot ulcres and their recurrence. N Engl J Med. 2017;376:2367–75.
4. Earwood J, et al. Septic arthritis: diagnosis and treatment. AFP. 2021;104(6):589–97.
5. Parvizi J, et al. The 2018 definition of periprosthetic hip and knee infection: an evidence-based and validated criteria. J Arthroplast. 2018;33:1309–14.
6. Edwards G, et al. What diagnostic strategies can help differentiate cellulitis from other causes of red legs in primary care? BMJ. 2020;368:m54. https://doi.org/10.1136/bmj.m54.
7. Swartz M. Cellulitis. N Engl J Med. 2004;350:904–12.
8. ☺☺☺Raff A, Kroshinsky D. Cellulitis. A review. JAMA. 2016;316(3):325–37.
9. Phoenix G, et al. Diagnosis and management of cellulitis. BMJ. 2012;345:e4955.
10. Raff A, et al. A predicrtive model for diagnosis of lower extremity cellulitis: a cross-sectional study. J Am Acad Dermatol. 2017;76:618–25.
11. Ezaldein H, et al. Risk stratification for cellulitis versus noncellulitic conditions of the lower extremity: a retrospective review of the NEW HAvUN criteria. Cutis. 2018;102:E8–E12.
12. Gunderson C. Cellulitis: definition, etiology, and clinical features. Am J Med. 2011;124:1113–22.
13. ☺Wall D, et al. A simple model to help distinguish necrotizing fasciitis from nonnecrotizing soft tissue infeciton. J Am Coll Surg. 2000;191:227–31.
14. ☺☺Stevens D, Bryant A. Necrotizing soft-tissue infections. N Engl J Med. 2017;377:2253–65.
15. Lancerotto L, et al. Nectrotizing fasciities: classification, diagnosis, and management. J Trauma. 2012;72:560–6.
16. Wong C, et al. The LRINEC (Laboratory Risk Indicator for Necrotizing Fasciitis) score: a tool for distinguishing necrotizing fasciitis from other soft tissue infections. Crit Care Med. 2004;32:1535–41.
17. Hussein Q, Anaya D. Necrotizing soft tissue infections. Crit Care Clin. 2013;29:795–806.
18. Armstrong DG, Tan TW, Boulton AJM et al. "Diabetic Foot Ulcers" JAMA 2023;330:62–75.
19. Mills JL, Conte MS, Armstrong DG et al. "The Society for Vascular Surgery lower extremity threatened limb classification system: Risk stratification based on Wound, Ischemia, and foot Infection (WIfI) J Vasc Surgery 2024;59:220–34.
20. van Reijen NS, Ponchant K, Ubbink DT, et al. "The prognostic value of the WIfI classifciation in patients with chronic limb threatening ischaemia: A systematic review and meta-analysis." Eur J Vasc Endovasc Surg 2019;58:362–71.

Inpatient Dermatology

23

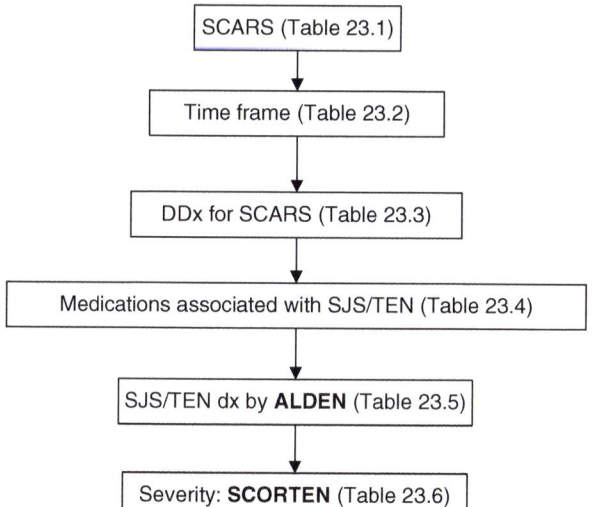

Exanthematous Drug Eruption or SCARS (Severe Cutaneous Adverse Reactions)

Table 23.1 SCARS

Fever
Mucous membrane involvement
Large blisters
Facial edema
Pustulosis
Visceral involvement

Duong et al. [1]

SJS/TEN/DRESS/AGEP

- T-cell mediated delayed hypersensivity reaction [1, 2]
- Distinction between SJS and TEN [3]

Table 23.2 SCAR interval and mortality

	Drug to SCAR interval	Mortality
SJS/TEN	4–28 days	10–40%
DRESS	2–6 weeks	1–10%
AGEP	1–11 days	1%

Duong et al. [1]

- 4–28 days between beginning of exposure and onset of reaction is the most suggestive timing for SJS/TEN (Mockenhaupt J Invest Derm [4])

Table 23.3 SCARS DDx

Large blisters		Fever Facial edema Eosinophils Visceral involvement	Fever pustulosis
No mucosal involvement	+ mucosal involvement	DRESS syndrome	AGEP
Fixed drug eruption	Skin detachment		
Linear IgA bullous dermatosis	<10% SJS 10–30% SJS-TEN 30% < TEN		

Duong et al. [1]

Table 23.4   Medications associated with SJS/TEN

Nevirapine
Lamotrigine
Carbamazepine
Phenytoin
Phenobarbital
Cotrimoxazole and other sulfonamides
Sulfasalazine
Allopurinol
Oxicam-NSAIDs
- Anti-infective sulfonamides are much higher risk than other antibiotics.
- Valpronic acid doesn't seem to be a major risk factor
- Sulfonamide-related diuretics and antidiabetics doesn't appear to be a risk.

Mockenhaupt et al. [4]

Table 23.5   ALDEN: algorithm of drug causality for epidermal necrolysis for SJS and TEN

Variable and point	
Variable	Point
Days from exposure to reaction	
1–4 days	1
5–28 days	3
29–56 days	2
>56 days	−1
Drug started after reaction	−3
Drug present or not	
Drug continued or stopped <×5 half-life	0
Drug stopped >×5 half-life but drug	−1
interaction possible	−3
Drug stopped >×5 half-life	
Pre-challenge/rechallenge	
No reaction to the same drug	−2
No known previous exposure	0
Other reaction after similar drug	1
SJS/TEN with similar drug	2
SJS/TEN with the same drug	4
Stopped	
Drug continued without harm	−2
Drug stopped or unknown	0
Type of drug	
No evidence of association	−1
Unknown	0
Several reports	1
Known low risk	2
Known high risk	3
Other cause is possible	−1
<0	Very unlikely
0–1	Unlikely
2–3	Possible
4–5	Probable
≥6	Very probable

Sassolas et al. [5]; Stern et al. [2]

Table 23.6 SCORTEN: severity score for TEN

Variable and point	
Variable	Point
Age ≥ 40	1
HR ≥ 120	1
Cancer/hematologic malignancy	1
Epidermal detachment >10% of BSA on day1	1
BUN>28 mg/dL	1
Glucose >252 mg/dL	1
Bicarbonate <20 mEq/L	1
Score and mortality (%)	
Total score	Mortality (%)
0–1	3.2
2	12.2
3	35.5
4	58.3
≥5	90.0

Bastuji-Garin et al. [6]; Schwartz et al. [7]

References

1. Duong T, et al. Severe cutanous adverse reactions to drugs. Lancet. 2017;390:1996–2011.
2. ☺ ☺ Stern R. Exanthematous drug eruptions. N Engl J Med. 2012;366:2492–501.
3. Bastuji-Garin S, et al. Clinical classification of cases of toxic epidermal necrolysis, Stevens-Johnson syndrome, and erythema multiforme. Arch Dermatol. 1993;129:92–6.
4. Mockenhaupt M, et al. Stevens-Johnson syndrome and toxic epidermal necrolysis: assessment of medication risks with emphasis on recently marketed drugs. The EuroSCAR-study. J Invest Derm. 2008;128:35–44.
5. Sassolas B, et al. ALDEN, an algorithm for assessment of drug causality in Stevens-Johnson syndrome and toxic epidermal necrolysis: comparison with case-control analysis. Clin Pharmacol Ther. 2010;88(1):60–8.
6. Bastuji-Garin S, et al. SCORETEN: a severity-of-illness score for toxic epidermal necrolysis. J Invest Dermatol. 2000;115:149–53.
7. Schwartz R, et al. Toxic epidermal necrolysis. Part II. Prognosis, sequelae, diagnosis, diffential diagnosis, prevention, and treatment. J Am Acad Dermatol. 2013;69:187.e181–16.

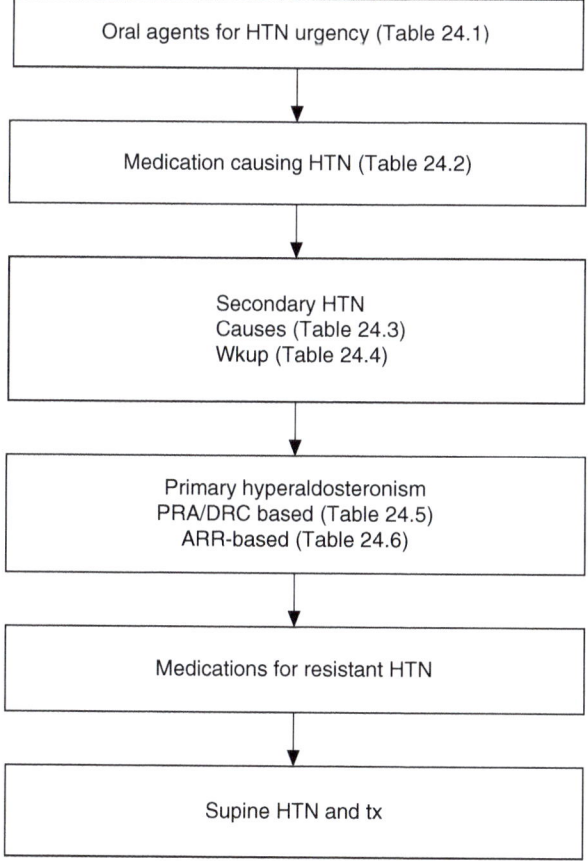

- Natural hx of BP: SBP, DBP, PP [1, 2]
- 'Guyton hypothesis' [3–5] and 'Laragh method' [6]
- Prothrombotic paradox [7]
- Oral agent for hypertensive urgency [8]
- Supine HTN and treatment [9]

Urgency vs Emergency
- No clear benefit to treat severe asymptomatic HTN (>180/110) up to 6 months [8, 10]
- Oral agents to work faster: clonidine, labetalol, captopril, prazosin [8]

Table 24.1 Oral agents

Meds	Dose
Clonidine	0.1–0.3 mg
Labetalol	200–400 mg
Captopril	25–50 mg
Prazosin	5–10 mg
Nitroglycerin 2% oint	1–2 inch

- There is no evidence that asymptomatic elevated BP will lead to end organ damage
- Normal BP for hospitalized patients is unknown [11]

Guidelines are not produced regularly anymore but the most recent one was JNC8 [12] as follows:

- BP goal: Age ≥ 60, <150/90, Age < 60, <140/90
- If nonblack, start with HCTZ, ACEI/ARB, CCB alone or in combination
- If black, start HCTZ, CCB alone or in combination
- CKD with/without DM, start with ACE/ARB
- As in BARBER-2 study [13] Black pts., with stage 2 or stage 1 with ASCVD>10% in 10 years should be on 2-medicines [14]

Table 24.2 Medications elevate BP

Category	Medications
Anticonvulsants	Carbamazepine
Antidepressants	MAOi
	SSRI/SNRI
	TCA
	Buspirone
Antipsychotics	Clozapine, thioridazine
Antiemetics	Metoclopramide, prochlorperazine
Hormones	Estrogen, steroid
Anti-inflammatory	NSAID
Anti-infectives	ketoconazole
Sympathomimetics	Decongestants
Illicit	Amphetamines, cocaine
Chemotherapy agents	
Calcineurin inhibitors	Cyclosporin, tacrolimus
Antineoplastic	Alkylating agents
	Paclitaxel
VEGF inhibitors	
Tyrosine kinase inhibitors	

Charles et al. [15]; Fay and Cohen [16]

Relevant facts to remember for hospitalized patients:

- ICH, DO NOT TREAT HTN unless SBP >220
- Ischemic stroke: Whelton et al. [17]
    - If BP < 220/110: do no harm
    - If BP > 220/110, LOWER BP 15% DURING FIRST 24 HOURS
    - If thrombolysis, SBP < 185, DBP <110 before thrombolysis and < 180/105 for first 24 hours after IV thrombolysis
    After 72 hours of CVA/TIA, >140/90, start meds aim <130/80
- Calcium channel blocker and diuretics would be a better choice than RAAS (ACEI or ARB) due to their property to decrease BP variability which is a RF for CVA. Beta-blocker should be avoided [18]

Secondary HTN

Table 24.3 Causes for secondary HTN

Causes	Prevalence (%)	diagnosis	Treatment
OSA	25–50	polysomnography	CPAP
Primary aldosteronism	8–20	Plasma renin, aldosterone	MRA, tumor resection
Renal artery stenosis	2–24	Renal doppler US	Revascularization in selected pt
Drug/alcohol induced	2–4	History/UTox	discontinuation
Renal parenchymal disease	1–2	Serum creatinine Renal US Renal Bx	Tx underlying causes

Whelton et al. [17];Vongpatanasin [19]

Table 24.4 Workup by age for secondary HTN

Age group	Child/ adolescent (<19 y/0)	Young adult (19–39 y/o)	Middle aged adult (40–64)	Older adults (≥65)
Etiologies	Renal parenchymal disease Coarctation of aorta	Thyroid dysfunction Renal artery stenosis due to fibromuscular dysplasia	OSA Hyperaldosteronism Cushing Pheochromocytoma	Renal artery stenosis due to atherosclerosis CKD
Workup	Urinalysis Renal US	TSH CT angiography	Renin/aldosterone TSH Sleep study 24 hr. Urine for cortisol, metanephrines	Renal artery doppler US

Charles et al. [15], Fig. 1

Primary Hyperaldosteronism

There are currently 2 ways to workup for primary hyperaldosteronism (PA): PRA/DRC and ARR

- PRA (plasma renin activity), DRC (direct renin concentration) and aldosterone level instead of ARR (Aldo-to-renin ratio) due to low se and sp. of ARR
- First measure plasma renin and serum aldosterone

Table 24.5 PRA, DRC based

PRA (ng/mL/h)	<1			1–20	20<
DRC (pg/mL)	<10			10–250	250<
Aldosterone (ng/dL)	<10	10–20	20<	Consider MRA	Consider renovascular disease
	MRA	Possible PA	Primary aldosteronism (PA)		

Byrd et al. [20]

Table 24.6 ARR-based

ARR (ng/mIU)	<20.6	20.6–45	45<
	PA unlikely	Consider repeat ARR	Adrenal CT, adrenal venous anatomy for adrenal vein sampling

Rossi [21]

Approach to Resistant HTN

Resistant HTN

- BP > 140/90 mmHg with hx of DM and/or CKD
- ≥ 3 antihypertnsive meds

Strategies for resistant HTN

1. Restrict sodium intake
2. Review nonprescription medications/supplements/Etoh use
3. If creatinine ≤1.5 mg/dl (or eGFR>30), continue HCTZ, if >1.5 (or eGFR≤30), use a loop diuretics
4. Investigate secondary HTN
5. Make sure 3 classes of meds are balanced
6. Strat MRA (spironolactone/eplerenone) if eGFR>30 (creatinine ≤1.5)
7. Additional meds if HR >80

Class		
1	Vasodilators	ACEI/ARB/DCCB
2	HR lowering agents	β-blockers/NDCCB
3	Diuretics	HCTZ/Loop/SGLT2i

Strategy	Meds
Combined α and β blocker	Carvedilol, labetalol
Dual CCB	DCCB + NDCCB
Centrally acting agent	Clonidine tab or patch
Direct vasodilators	Hydralazine, minoxidil

8. If HR < 60, avoid above and add α-blocker [19, 22]

- Even if eGFR<30, after add loop to HCTZ and if BP is not at goal, you can add MRA but if potassium >5.5, then add potassium-binding polymer [16]
- After PATHWAY-2 study [23], MRA became preferred fourth medication. And AMBER study [24] used Patiromer to facilitate the use of spironolactone for resistant HTN.
- fifth meds would be to against increased sympathetic tone, β-, α-blockers or central α- agonist
- Based on the current best knowledge, PATHWAY-2 and AMBER, the emerging strategy for resistant HTN [25] is as follows:

Emerging Therapy for Resistant HTN
1. MRAs
2. Potassium binders (patiromer) to control hyperkalemia due to MRA
3. Carotid baroreceptor activation therapy
4. Catheter-based renal nerve denervation

Supine HTN
- Supine HTN affect 50% of patients with neurogenic orthostatic hypotension patient and antihypertensives make it worse [26].
- Δ HR/ Δ mmHg >0.5 has high sensitivity and specificity for non-neurogenic OH [9, 26].
- Nocturnal supine HTN leads to nocturnal diuresis and relative volume depletion and which leads to worsening of daytime OH [9].
- Avoid bed rest and do PT is the first line tx for OH and recommends sleeping in head up tilt to reduce nocturnal diuresis. (also Goldstein and Sharabi [27] in syncope section OH)
- Head elevation reduces nocturnal diuresis [9]
- Treatment strategy of supine HTN [28] ONLY QHS
- Treatment of supine HTN will often exacerbates OH: prefers ACEI/ARB/Ca blocker over central sympatholytics or alpha blocker [9]
- Avoid diuretics in elderly with supine HTN and pressure diuresis [9]

Meds	Mechanism of action	Dose
Captopril	ACEI	25 mg QHS
Clonidine	Central α-2 agonist	0.2 mg with evening meal
Hydralazine	Peripheral smooth muscle relaxant	10–25 mg QHS
Losartan	Angiotensin II receptor antagonist	50 mg QHD
Nitroglycerine patch	vasodilator	0.1 mg/h QHS

References

1. ☺ ☺ Safar M, et al. Current perspectives on arterial stiffness and pulse pressure in hypertension and cardiovascular diseases. Circulation. 2003;107:2864–9.
2. ☺ ☺ ☺ O'Rourke M, Seward J. Central arterial pressure and arterial pressure pulse: new views entering the second century after Korotkov. Mayo Clin Proc. 2006;81:1057–68.
3. ☺ ☺ ☺ Palmer BF. Renal dysfunction complicating the treatment of hypertension. New Engl J Med. 2002;347:1256–61.
4. ☺ Johnson R, et al. Subtle acquired renal injury as a mechanism of salt-sensitive hypertension. N Engl J Med. 2002;346:913–23.
5. ☺ ☺ Adrogue H, Madias N. Sodium and potassium in the pathogenesis of hypertension. Ibid. 2007;356:1966–78.
6. Laragh J, Sealey J. The plasma renin test reveals the contribution of body sodium-volume content (V) and renin-angiotensin (R) vasocontriction to long-term blood pressure. Am J Hypertension. 2011;24(11):1164–80.
7. Messerli F, et al. Essential hypertension. Lancet. 2007;370:591–603.
8. ☺ ☺ ☺ Peixoto A. Acute severe hypertension. N Engl J Med. 2019;381:1843–52.
9. ☺ ☺ Wahba A, et al. Management of orthostatic hpotension in the hospitalized patient: a narrative review. Am J Med. 2022;135:24–31.
10. Gauer R. Severe asymptomatic hypertension: evaluation and treatment. AFP. 2017;95(8):492–500.
11. Stanistreet B, et al. An evidence-based review of elevated blood pressure for the inpatient. Am J Med. 2020;133:165–9.
12. ☺ ☺ ☺ James P, et al. 2014 Evidence-based guideline for the management of high blood pressure in adults. Report from the Panel Members Appointed to the Eighth Joint National Committee (JNC 8). JAMA. 2014;311(5):507–20.
13. Victor R, et al. Effectiveness of a barber-based intervention for improving hyptension control in black men. The BARBER-1 study: a cluster randomized trial. Arch Intern M. 2011;171(4):342–50.
14. Sulaica E, et al. A review of hypertension management in black male patients. Mayo Clin Proc. 2020;95(9):1955–63.
15. ☺ ☺ ☺ Charles L, et al. Secondary hypertension: discovering the underlying cause. AFP. 2017;96(7):453–61.
16. Fay K, Cohen D. Resistant hypertension in people with CKD: A review. Am J Kidney Dis. 2021;77(1):110–21.
17. ☺ ☺ ☺ Whelton P, et al. 2017 ACC/AHA/AAPA/ABC/ACPM/AGS/APhA/ASH/ASPC/NMA/PCNA guideline for the prevention, detection, evaluation, and management of high blood pressure in adults: executive summary. J Am Coll Cardiol. 2018;71(19):2199–269.
18. Rothwell P, et al. Stroke care 1. Medical treatment in acute and long-term secondary prevention after transient ischaemic attack and ischaemic stroke. Lancet. 2011;377:1681–92.
19. ☺ ☺ Vongpatanasin W. Resistant hypertension. A review of diagnosis and management. JAMA. 2014;311(21):2216–24.
20. Byrd J, et al. Primary aldosteronism. Practical approach to diagnosis and management. Circulation. 2018;138:823–35.
21. Rossi G. Primary aldosteronism. J Am Coll Cardiol. 2019;74:2799–811.
22. ☺ ☺ ☺ Moser M, Setaro J. Resistant or difficult -to-control hypertension. N Engl J Med. 2006;355:385–92.
23. Williams B, et al. Spironolactone versus placebo, bisoprolol, and doxazosin to determine the optimal treatment for drug-resistant hypertension (PATHWAY-2): a randomised, double-blind, crossover trial. Lancet. 2015;386:2059–68.

24. Agarwal R, et al. Patiromer versus placebo to enable spironolactone use in patients with resistant hypertension and chronic kidney disease (AMBER): a phase 2, randomised, double-blind, placebo-controlled trial. Ibid. 2019;394:1540–50.
25. Epstein M, Duprez D. Resistant hypertension and the pivotal role for mineralcorticoid receptor antagonists: a clinical update 2016. Am J Med. 2016;129:661–6.
26. Kim M, Farrell J. Orthostatic hypotension: a practical approach. AFP. 2022;105(1):39–49.
27. Goldstein D, Sharabi Y. Neurogenic orthostatic hypotension: a pathophsiological approach. Circulation. 2009;119:139–46.
28. Gibbons C, et al. The recommendations of a consensus panel for the screening, diagnosis, and treatment of neurogenic orthostatic hypotension and associated supine hypertension. J Neurol. 2017;264:1567–82.

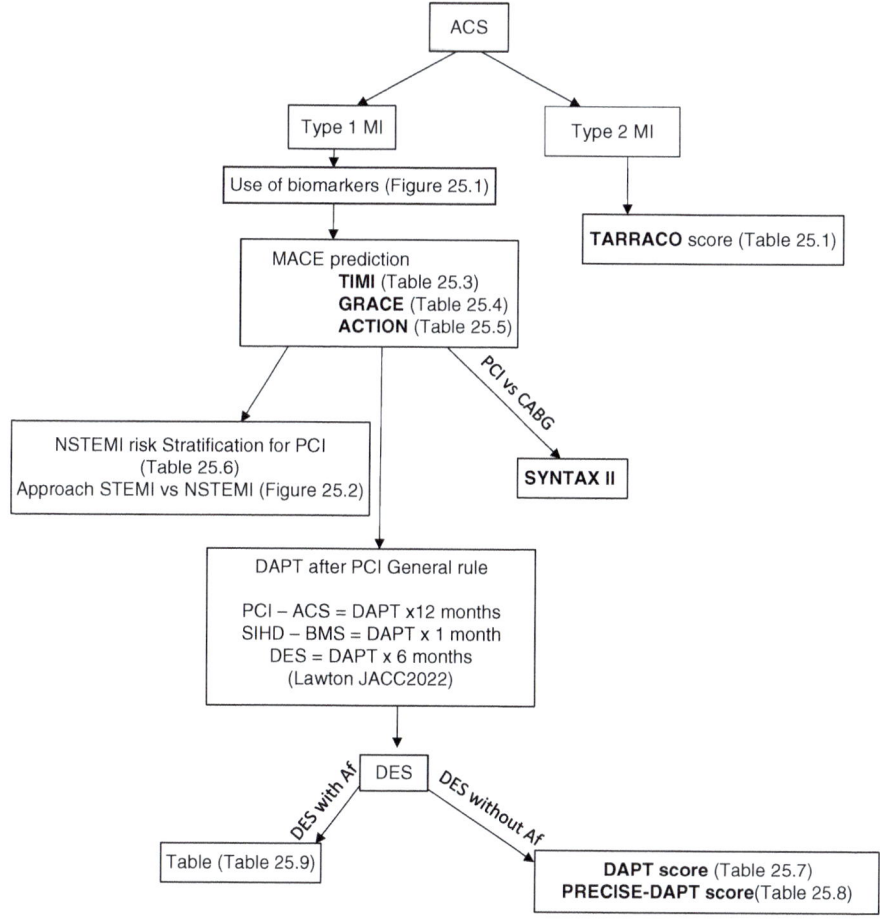

M. J. Morikawa, *The Inpatient Medicine Handbook*,
https://doi.org/10.1007/978-3-032-08398-2_25

Type 2 MI
- 49% mortality in 2 years [1]

Table 25.1 TARRACO risk score

Variable	Points
Age	
<70	0
70–79	1
80≤	3
HTN	2
Absence of chest pain	2
Dyspnea	2
Anemia (Hb < 13 in male, <12 in female)	3
Troponin >5URL	1

Risk category	Points
Low	0–6
High	7–13

Event rate (all-cause mortality, CHF readmission or AMI) in 180 days	
Risk category	Event rate (%)
Low	10.2
High	28.6

Cediel et al. [2]

Type 1 MI
- Chest pain r/o using 0- and 3-hour Troponin

Fig. 25.1 Dx by biomarkers

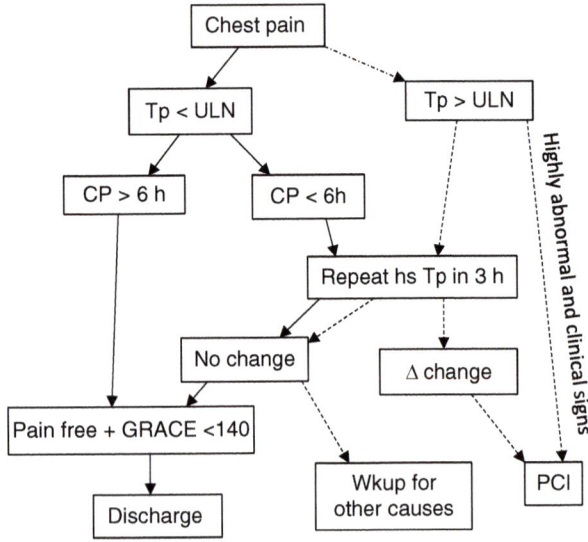

Table 25.2 Use of troponin I

• 0- and 1- hour R/I and R/O algorithm with Tp I for suspected NSTEMI		
0 h < 2 ng/L or 0 h < 5 ng/L and Δ0–1 h < 2 ng/L	Other	0 h ≥ 52 ng/L or Δ 0–1 h ≥ 6 ng/L
R/O	Observation	R/I

Hollander et al. [3]

Outcome Prediction

Table 25.3 TIMI score

• 14-day MACE prediction	
TIMI risk items	
Age ≥ 65	
At least 3 risk factors for CAD (HTN, Hypercholesterol, DM, SMK)	
Significant coronary stenosis (stenosis ≥50%)	
ST deviation	
Severe anginal symptoms (≥2 anginal events in last 24 hr)	
Use of ASA in last 7 days	
Elevated serum cardiac markers	
Outcome (%)	
TIMI score	Outcome
0/1	4.7
2	8.3
3	13.2
4	19.9
5	26.2
6/7	40.9

Antman et al. [4]

Table 25.4 GRACE score

• Estimates 6-month mortality after ACS admission	
Variable	Point
Age	
≤29	0
30–39	0
40–49	18
50–59	36
60–69	55
70–79	73
80–89	91
≥90	100
Hx of CHF	24
Hx of MI	12

(continued)

Table 25.4 (continued)

• Estimates 6-month mortality after ACS admission	
Variable	Point
Resting HR beats/min	
≤49.9	0
50–69.9	3
70–89.9	9
90–109.9	14
110–149.9	23
150–199.0	35
≥200	43
SBP mmHg	
≤79.9	24
80–99.9	22
100–119.9	18
120–139.9	14
140–159.9	10
160–199.9	4
≥200	0
ST depression	11
Initial serum creatinine mg/dL	
0–0.39	1
0.4–0.79	3
0.8–1.19	5
1.2–1.59	7
1.6–1.99	9
2–3.99	15
≥4	20
Elevated cardiac enzymes	15
No in-hospital PCI	14

Eagle and Lim [5]

• Score > 140 correlates with >10% mortality in 6 months

Long-term consequences of GRACE score

• Discharge GRACE score was valid at 2-year post discharge.
• Low ≤108; intermediate 109–140; high >140 and outcome
• Score > 140 correlates with >25% mortality in 2 years [6]

Table 25.5 ACTION

In-hospital mortality prediction	
Variables and points	
Variable	Points
Age	
<40	0
40–49	3
50–59	7
60–69	9
70–79	13
80–89	17
90<	20
SBP	
200<	0
181–200	3
171–180	5
161–170	7
151–160	9
131–150	11
121–130	13
111–120	15
91–110	16
≤90	19
CrCl	
95<	0
60–90	4
45–60	8
30–45	11
<30 or HD	15
Cardiac arrest	
No	0
Yes	14
Shock	
No	0
Yes	13
Heart rate	
<40	0
41–60	1
61–70	2
71–80	3
81–100	4
101–110	5
111–130	7
131–150	8
150<	9
Heart failure	
No	0
Yes	5

(continued)

Table 25.5 (continued)

• In-hospital mortality prediction	
Variables and points	
Variable	Points
STEMI	
No	0
Yes	5
Troponin	
<1	0
1–10	0
20–20	1
20–30	2
30<	3

Points	In-hospital mortality (%)
<30	0.4
30–39	1.7
40–49	5.5
50–59	18.5
59<	49.5

McNamara et al. [7]

SYNTAX II score can provide 4-year mortality with either CABG vs PCI

• Variables for this scoring is age, CrCl, LVEF, left main disease or not, sex, hx of COPD and PAD [8].

Risk Stratification for PCI

Table 25.6 risk stratification for NSTEMI

	Invasive intervention			Ischemia-guided intervention
Timing	< 2 hr	<24 hr	25–72 hr	>72 hr
Indication	Refractory angina New onset HF New/worsening MR Recurrent angina refractory to medical tx	GRACE>140 Rising troponin New ST depression	GRACE 109–140 TIMI ≥2 EF < 40% Postinfarction angina DM CKD Prior CABG Recent PCI (<6 mo)	TIMI 0 or 1 Troponin negative

Anderson and Morrow [9]

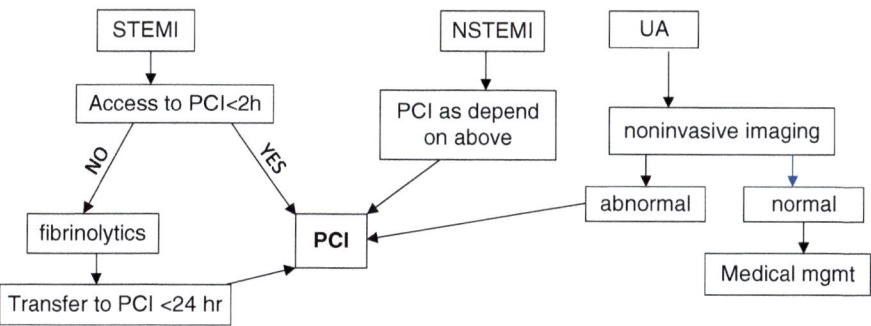

Fig. 25.2 Approach with STEMI vs NSTEMI (Bhatt et al. [10])

Approach for DAPT After PCI

Table 25.7 DAPT score

• Score ≥ 2 would benefit continue DAPT over 1 year	
Variable	Point
Age	
≥75	−2
65–75	−1
<65	0
SMK	1
DM	1
MI at presentation	1
Prior PCI or MI	1
Paclitaxel-eluting stent	1
Stent diameter <3 mm	1
Vein graft stent	2
CHF or LVEF<30%	2

Yeh et al. [11]

Table 25.8 PRECISE-DAPT score

• Hb, Age, Ccr, WBC and prior bleed		
• 1 year bleeding risk prediction		
• ≥25 considered as higher risk and recommend shorter course of DAPT tx		
DAPT duration after DES: DAPT algorithm based on 2 risk scores: DAPT and PRECISE-DAPT [12]		
	PRECISE-DAPT score	
	<25	≥25
SCAD	6 months	3 months
ACS	DAPT score < 2 then 12 months	6 months
	DAPT score ≥ 2 up to 18 months	

Costa et al. [13]

Table 25.9 Anticoagulation/antiplatelet after PCI for patients with Af

High ischemic risk	Average risk	High bleeding risk
Triple (DOAC + DAPT) × 1 month	Triple × 1 week (or hospital stay)	Triple × 1 week (or hospital stay)
DOAC + clopidogrel × 12 months	DOAC + clopidogrel × 12 months	DOAC + clopidogrel × 6 months
Then DOAC	Then DOAC	Then DOAC

Capodanno et al. [14]; Bergmark et al. [15]

References

1. Saaby L, et al. Mortality rates in type 2 myocardial infarction: observations from an unselected hospital cohort. Am J Med. 2014;127:295–302.
2. Cediel G, et al. Risk estimation in type 2 myocardial infarction and myocardial injury: the TARRACO risk score. Ibid. 2019;132:217–26.
3. ☺ ☺ Hollander J, et al. State-of-the-art evaluation of emergency department patients presenting with potential acute coronary syndrome. Circulation. 2016;134:547–64.
4. Antman E, et al. The TIMI risk score for unstable angina/non-ST elevation MI. A method for prognostication and therapeutic decision making. JAMA. 2000;284:835–42.
5. Eagle K, Lim M. A validated prediction model for all forms of acute coronary syndrome. Estimating the risk of 6-month postdischarge death in an international registry. Ibid. 2004;291:2727–33.
6. Alnasser S, et al. Late consequences of acute coronary syndromes: Global Registry of Acute Coronary Events (GRACE) follow-up. Am J Med. 2015;128:766–75.
7. McNamara R, et al. Pedicting in-hospital mortality in patients with acute myocardial infarction. J Am Coll Cardiol. 2016;68:626–35.
8. Farooq V, et al. Anatomical and clinical characteristics to guide decision making between coronary artery bypass surgery and percutaneous coronary intevention for individual patients: development and validation of SYNTAX score II. Lancet. 2013;381:639–50.
9. ☺ ☺ ☺ Anderson J, Morrow D. Acute myocardial infarction. N Engl J Med. 2017;376:2053–64.
10. Bhatt D, et al. Diagnosis and treatment of acute coronary syndromes. A review. JAMA. 2022;327(7):662–75.

11. Yeh R, et al. Development and validation of a prediction rule for benefit and harm of dual antiplatelet therapy beyond 1 year after precutanous coronary intervention. Ibid. 2016;315(16):1735–49.

12. ☺ ☺ ☺ Torrado J, et al. Restenosis, stent thrombosis, and bleeding complications. Navigating between Scylla and Charybdis. J Am Coll Cardiol. 2018;71:1676–95.

13. Costa F, et al. Derivation and validation of the predicting bleeding complications in patients undergoing stent implantation and subsequent dual antiplatelet therapy (PRECISE-DAPT) score, a pooled analysis of individual-patient datasets from clinical trials. Lancet. 2017;389:1025–34.

14. Capodanno D, Huber K, Mehran R, et al. "Management of antithrombotic therapy in atrial fibrillation patients undergoing PCI." J Am Coll Cardiol. 2019;74:83–99.

15. Bergmark B, et al. Acute coronary syndromes. Ibid. 2022;399:1347–58.

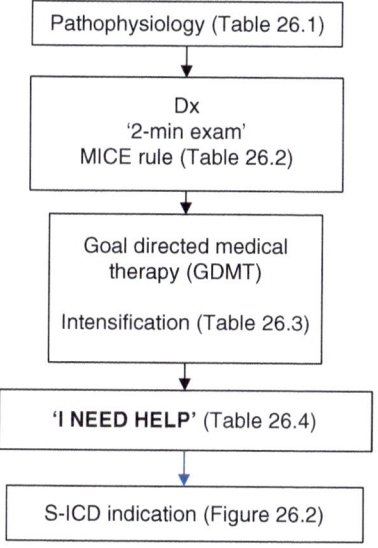

Fig. 26.1 Workflow of HFrEF

M. J. Morikawa, *The Inpatient Medicine Handbook*,
https://doi.org/10.1007/978-3-032-08398-2_26

Table 26.1 Pathophysiology

Neurohormonal	Schrier and Abraham [1]McMurray and Pfeffer [2]
Aldosterone	Weber [3] Urine Na/K ratio
Afterload mismatch	Cotter et al. [4]
Metabolic	Neubauer [5]Ashrafian et al. [6]
Vasopeptide inhibition	Palmer and Clegg [7]Packer and McMurray [8]Packer [9]
"2-minutes assessment of hemodynamic profile" (see ADHF section Fig. 26.1) Based on perfusion (warm or cold) and filling pressure (dry or wet)	

Dx: Nohria et al. [10]

Table 26.2 MICE rule

Male, infarction, crepitations, edema rule If patient present symptoms such as dyspnea for HF, refer straight to 2DEcho if the patients have any of the following: hx of MI, or basal crackles or male with ankle edema. Otherwise, carry out BNP and refer 2Decho depending on the result.

Roalfe et al. [11]

Diagnostic procedures and biomarkers:

- Abnormal EKG, BNP ≥ 35 pg/mL, or NT-pro-BNP ≥125 pg/mL then obtain 2D Echo [12]
- "sST2 as the HbA1c of HF" [13]
- R/O Dx of HF if BNP <35 pg/mL or NT-proBNP <125 pg/mL [14]

CXR: In ADHERE sample, 20% of patients with ADHF had negative CXR [15].

Tx: GDMT

4 meds with target dosing for HFrEF.

Beta-blocker (BB).
ARNI or ACEI/ARB.
MRA
SGLT2 inhibitor (SGLT2i).

Initiation of GDMT.

SBP > 100	SBP <100
ARNI	ACEI/ARB
+	+
Diuretics	Diuretics

Evaluate 24–48 hours.

Minimal congestion	Continued congestion SBP >100
Add BB	Add SGLT2i
+	
As long as stable renal function add MRA	

Discharge

Ensure to be on all 4 classes
HR goal <70
SBP 100–130

- Higher priority goes to BB and ARNI due to greatest mortality benefit (Dimza et al. [18])

If no improvement, or persistent symptoms, try 'intensification of tx'.

Table 26.3 Intensification of tx

If on ACEI/ARB	Switch to ARNI
If GFR > 30 and K < 5.0	Add MRA
If HR ≥ 70 in NSR and on maximally tolerated β-blocker	Add ivabradine
African American patients on ARNI/β-blocker/MRA and continued symptoms	Isosorbide dinitrate + hydralazine

Murphy et al. [14]

Table 26.4 I NEED HELP.

Worsening symptoms then "I NEED HELP" to refer advanced HF specialist	
I	IV inotropes
N	NYHA IIIB/IV symptoms or persistently elevated BNP
E	End-organ dysfunction
E	EF ≤ 35%
D	Defibrillator shocks
H	Hospitalization for HF ≥2 times in 12 months
E	Edema despite diuretics
L	Low BP or high HR
P	Progressive intolerance or step-down of GDMT

Murphy et al. [14]

Device therapy and device selection [16].

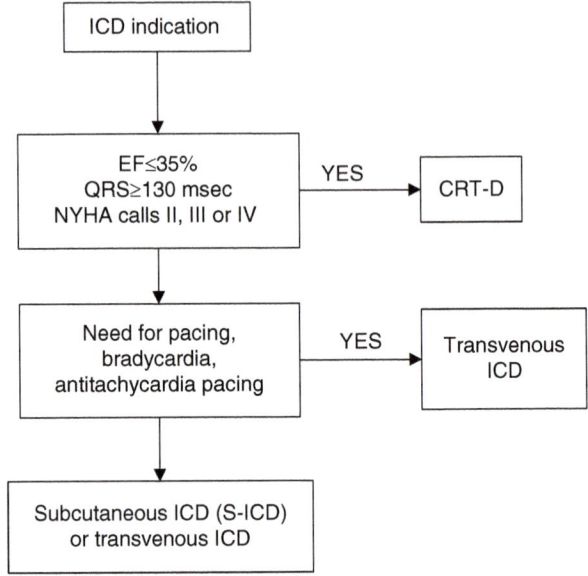

Fig. 26.2 Device selection

Strong indication of S-ICD.

Young age
Primary prevention
Poor vascular access
Previous infection
Infection risk (mechanical valves, DM, renal dysfunction)

Newer devices [17] are coming.

References

1. Schrier R, Abraham W. Hormones and hemodynamics in heart failure. N Engl J Med. 1999;341:577–86.
2. McMurray J, Pfeffer MA. New therapeutic options in congestive heart failure. Part II. Circulation. 2002;105:2223–8.
3. Weber KT. Aldosterone in congestive heart failure. N Engl J Med. 2001;345:1689–97.
4. Cotter G, et al. Acute heart failure: a novel approach to its pathogenesis and treatment. Eur J Heart Failure. 2002;4:227–34.
5. Neubauer S. The failing heart-an engine out of fuel. N Engl J Med. 2007;356:1140–51.
6. Ashrafian H, et al. Metabolic mechanisms in heart failure. Circulation. 2007;116:434–48.
7. Palmer B, Clegg D. An emerging role of natriuretic peptides: igniting the fat furnace to fuel and warm the heart. Mayo Clin Proc. 2015;90(12):1666–78.

8. Packer M, McMurray J. Importance of endogenous compensatory vasoactive peptides in broadening the effects of inhibitors of the renin-angiotensin system for the treatment of heart failure. Lancet. 2017;389:1831–40.

9. Packer M. Leptin-aldosterone-Neprilysin axis. Circulation. 2018;137:1614–31.

10. ☺Nohria A, et al. medical management of advanced heart failure. JAMA. 2002;287:628–40.

11. Roalfe A, et al. Development and intitial validation of a simple clinical decision tool to predict the presence of heart failure in primary care: the MICE (male, infraction, Crepitations, edema) rule. Eur J Heart Fail. 2012;14:1000–8.

12. Metra M, Teerlink J. Heart failure. Lancet. 2017;390:1981–95.

13. Wettersten N, Maisel A. Biomarkers for heart failure: an update for practitioners of internal medicine. Am J Med. 2016;129:560–7.

14. ☺☺☺Murphy S, et al. Heart failure with reduced ejection fraction. A review. JAMA. 2020;324(5):488–504.

15. Collins S, Lindsell C. Prevalence of negative chest radiography results in the emergency department patient with decompensated heart failure. Ann Emerg Med. 2006;47:13–8.

16. Al-Khatib S, et al. Defibrillators. Selecting the right device for the right patient. Circulation. 2016;134:1390–404.

17. Fudim M, et al. Device therapy in chronic heart failure. J Am Coll Cardiol. 2021;78:931–56.

18. Dimza M, Kurup V, Canha C, et al. "Pharmacological therapy optimization for heart failure: A practical guide for the internist." Am J Med. 2023;136:745–52.

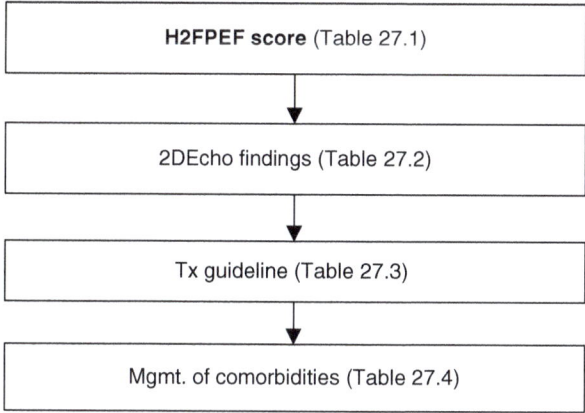

EPI:
- Older, female (62%), HTN in ADHERE registry [1]
- HFpEF has high mortality after hospitalization, 65% mortality in 5 years [2]
- Annual death rate was 5.2% in I-PRESERVE HFpEF cohort [3]
- Olmstead County cohort, 47% of CHF was HFpEF and survival was slightly better than HFrEF [4].

PATH
Protein kinase G may play a role in HFpEF [5].
Role of ROS and PKG [6].
Impaired myocardial relaxation and stiffness [7].

Dx of HFpEF: H2FPEF score or HFA-PEFF score.

Table 27.1 H2FPEF score

	Variable	Points
• Predict the diagnosis of HFpEF among patients with dyspnea on exertion		
• Score > 5 is diagnostic of HFpEF [8]		
H2	Heavy BMI > 30	2
	HTN: ≥2 antihypertensive meds	1
F	Atrial Fibrillation: paroxysmal or persistent	3
P	Pulmonary HTN PASP >35 mmHg	1
E	Elder: age > 60	1
F	Filling pressure E/e' > 9	1

Reddy et al. [9]

HFA-PEFF score

	Functional	Morphological	Biomarker (Sinus rhythm)	Biomarker (Af)
Major criteria (2 points)	Septal e' < 7 cm/s or lateral e' < 10 cm/s Average E/e' ≥ 15 TR velocity > 2.8 m/s	LA volume index >34 mL/m² LV mass index ≥149/122 g/m² and relative wall thickness > 0.42	NT-proBNP> 220 pg/ml BNP > 80 pg/ml	NT-proBNP>660 pg/ml BNP > 240 pg/ml
Minor criteria (1 point)	Average E/e'9–14 global longitudinal strain <16%	LAVI 29–34 LVMI>115/95 RWT > 0.42 LV wall thickness ≥ 12 mm	NT-proBNP 125–220 pg/ml BNP 35–80 pg/ml	NT-proBNP 365–660 pg/ml BNP 105–240 pg/ml

• Score ≥ 5 HFpEF
• 2–4 points diastolic stress test or invasive hemodynamic measures

Pieske et al. [10]

Scores and Diagnosis

	Low probability Unlikely HFpEF	Intermediate probability Further testing	High probability Likely HFpEF
H2FPEF score	0–1	2–5	6–9
HFA-PEFF score	0–1	2–4	5–6

DX 2DEcho Findings

1. LA volume
2. MIV
3. TDI

Table 27.2 MIV (Mitral Inflow Velocity) pattern in HFpEF

	Normal	Mild dysfunction impaired relaxation	Moderate pseudonormal	Severe restrictive
LV relaxation	Normal	Impaired	impaired	Impaired
LV compliance	Normal	↓	↓↓	↓↓↓
LA pressure	Normal	↑	↑↑	↑↑↑
E:A form	E > A	E < A	E > A	E> > A

Aurigemma and Gaasch [11]

Echo def [12–15].

Table 27.3 Treatment approach

1. Once HFpEF is confirmed, start SGLT2i
2. Assess volume overload,
3. If yes, add diuretics
4. Then treat comorbidities

Borlaug et al. [15]

Table 27.4 HFpEF comorbidities mgmt

Comorbidity	Mgmt
AF	Rate vs rhythm guided by symptoms
	BB or NDCCB (avoid aggressive rate control due to low SV)
	Anticoagulation
HTN	<130/80
	Diuretics, ARNI, ARB, MRA
OSA	Sleep study
	Weight loss
CAD	Medical mgmt
Obesity	Weight loss
	Ssemaglutide
T2DM	A1c < 7–7.5
	SGLT2i first, GLP1 if obesity
CKD	RAAS inhibitors and SGLT2i
	ARNI if eGFR>30
	SGLT2i if eGFR≥20

Kittleson et al. [8]

References

1. Whellan D, Harrington C. Diastolic heart failure and continuous hemodynamic monitoring. Am Heart J. 2007;153:S6–S11.
2. Shah S, Gheorghiade M. Heart failure with preserved ejection fraction: treat now by treating comorbidities. JAMA. 2008;300:431–3.
3. Udelson J. Heart failure with preserved ejection fraction. Circulation. 2011;124:e540–3.
4. ☺Owan T, et al. Trends in prevalence and outcome of heart failure with preserved ejection fraction. N Engl J Med. 2006;355:251–9.
5. Lyle M, Brozovich F. HFpEF, a disease of the vasculature; a closer look at the other half. Mayo Clin Proc. 2018;93(9):1305–14.
6. Paulus W, Tschope C. A novel paradigm for heart failure with preserved ejection fraction. J Am Coll Cardiol. 2013;62(4):263–71.
7. Oren O, Goldberg S. Heart failure with preserved ejection fraction: diagnosis and management. Am J Med. 2017;130:510–6.
8. ☺ ☺ ☺Kittleson M, et al. 2023 ACC expert consensus decision pathway on management of heart failure with preserved ejection fraction. J Am Coll Cardiol. 2023;81(18):1835–78.
9. ☺ ☺Reddy Y, et al. A simple, evidence-based approach to help guide diagnosis of heart failure with preserved ejection fraction. Circulation. 2018;138:861–70.
10. Pieske B, et al. How to diagnose heart failure with preserved ejection fraction: the HFA-PEFF diagnostic algorithm: a consensus recommendation from the Heart Failure Association (HFA) of the European Society of Cardiology (ESC). Eur Heart J. 2019;40:3297–317.
11. Aurigemma G, Gaasch W. Diastolic heart failure. N Engl J Med. 2004;351:1097–105.
12. Oghlakian G, et al. Treatment of heart failure with preserved ejection fraction: have we been pursuing the wrong paradigm? Mayo Clin Proc. 2011;86(6):531–9.
13. Paulus W, et al. How to diagnose diastolic heart failure: a consensus statement on the diagnosis of heart failure with normal left ventricular ejection fraction by the Heart Failure and Echocardiography Associations of the European Society of Cardiology. Eur Heart J. 2007;28:2539–50.
14. Redfield M, et al. Burden of systolic and diastolic ventricular dysfunction in the community. JAMA. 2003;289:194–202.
15. Borlaug B, et al. Heart failure with preserved ejection fraction. J Am Coll Cardiol. 2023;81:1810–34.

Acutely Decompensated Heart Failure (ADHF)

28

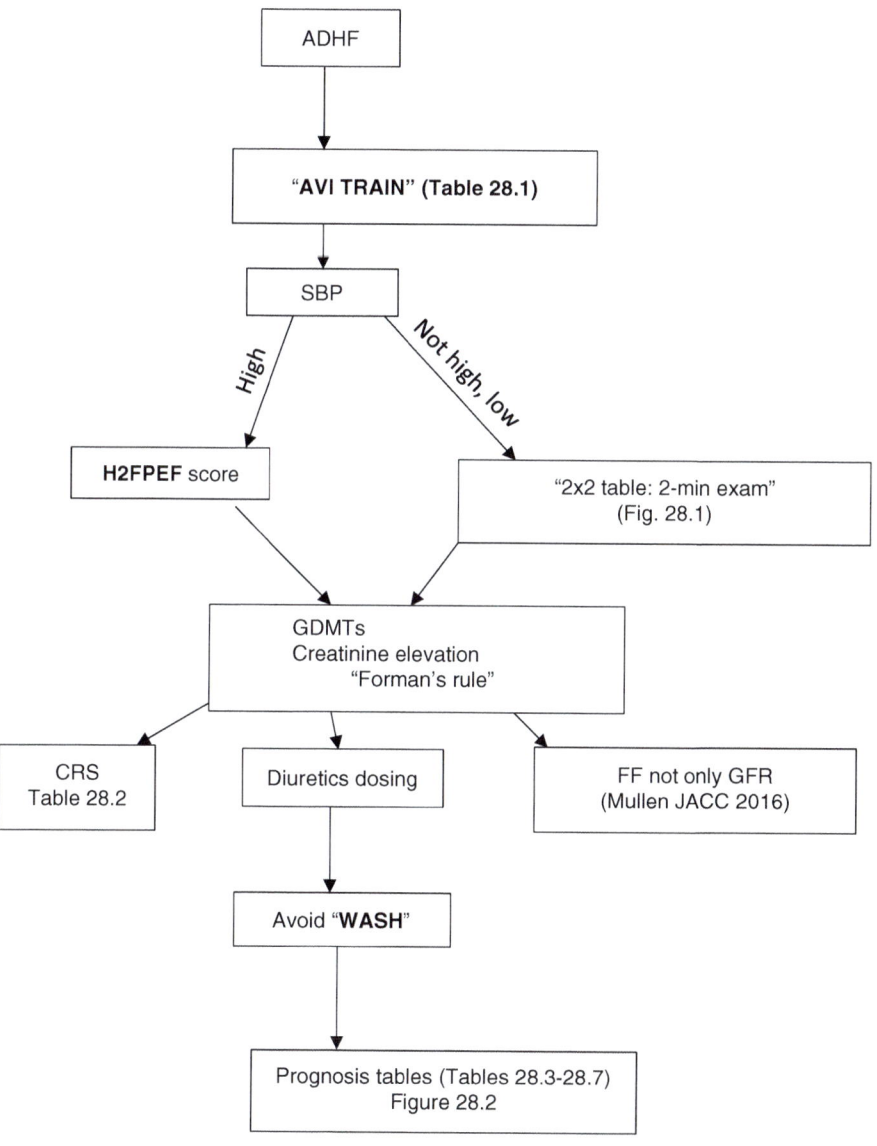

© The Author(s), under exclusive license to Springer Nature Switzerland AG 2025

M. J. Morikawa, *The Inpatient Medicine Handbook*,

https://doi.org/10.1007/978-3-032-08398-2_28

Pathophysiology: 2 pathways in ADHF [1].

Cardiac pathway	Vascular pathway
Low cardiac contractility	Increased vascular resistance
Fluid accumulation	Increased vascular stiffness
Renal impairment	Acute afterload mismatch
Pulmonary edema	Pulmonary edema

Etiology

Table 28.1 AVI TRAIN

	Etiologies
A	Arrythmias (Af is the most common)
V	Valvular (worsening of MR)
I	Infection
T	Thyroid issue
R	Renal problems
A	Anemia
I	Ischemia
N	Non-compliance (medication and/or diet)

Kittleson and Kobashigawa [2]

Assessment

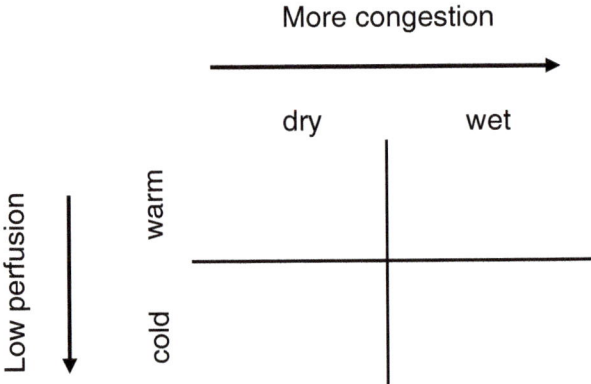

Fig. 28.1

"2 × 2 table"

Signs of poor perfusion	Signs of congestion
Narrow pulse pressure	Orthopnea
Cool extremities	JVD
Obtunded	Edema
Worsening renal function	Ascites
	Crackle (not specific)
	Abdo-jugular reflex

Kapoor and Perazellas [3]; Stevenson [4]; Hollenberg et al. [5]

Avoid 'WASH'

- 25% patients for ADHF admissions were 'wet and sent home' [6]
- The most common reasons in academic center were renal dysfunction

Cardiorenal Syndrome

Table 28.2 CRS classification [7]

Type 1	Type 2	Type 3	Type 4	Type 5
Acute primary cardiac affect renal	Chronic primary cardiac affect renal	Acute renal affects cardiac	Chronic renal affects cardiac	Secondary CRS

Approach to refractory CRS [8].

- Diuretic algorithm used in CARRESS-HF and AVOID-HF trials (Jentzer JACC 2020)

(See the table in Diuretic section)

Prognosis
Clinical assessment predicts outcome

- Clinical congestion at discharge predicts readmission and mortality [9]
- Heart failure score (symptoms) also correlates with mortality in MOST trial cohort [10]

Table 28.3 Composite congestion score (CCS)

	0	1	2	3
Orthopnea	None	Seldom	Frequent	Continuous
JVD (cm)	≤6	6–9	10–15	≥15
Pedal edema	None/trace	slight	moderate	marked

All-cause mortality by CCS	
Score	Mortality (%)
0	19.1
1	24.8
2	25.1
3–9	42.8

Table 28.4 1-year mortality based on clinical class

• ESC-EORP-HFA HF registry cohort [11]				
	Dry-warm	Wet-warm	Dry-cold	Wet-cold
1-year mortality (%)	12.1	22.6	28.0	26.4

Table 28.5 In-house mortality prediction

• Based on ADHERE registry			
• 3 RFs: BUN, Creatinine, SBP on admission [12]			
3 risk factor combination and in-house mortality (%)			
BUN≥43 mg/dL	SBP <115 mmHg	Serum creatinine ≥2.75 mg/dL	In-house mortality (%)
−	−		1.8
−	+		4.3
+	−		7.9
+	+	−	14.2
+	+	+	26.5

Table 28.6 EHMRG score (Emergency Heart Failure Mortality Risk Grade)

• 7-day mortality	
Variables and point	
Variable	Point
Age	2 × age
Transported by EMS	60
SBP mmHg	−1 × SBP
HR	1 × HR
Pox (%)	−2 × Pox
Creatinine (mg/dL)	20 × creatinine
Potassium	
4.0–4.5	0
≥4.6	30
≤3.9	5
Troponin elevation	60
Active cancer	45
Metolazone at home	60
Adjustment factor	12
Total points and 7-day mortality (%)	
Points	Mortality
≤−49.1	0.5
−49.0 to −15.9	0.3
−15.8 to 17.9	0.7
18.0 to 56.5	2.1
56.6 to 89.3	3.3
≥89.4	8.5

Lee et al. [13]

"When kidney fails, HF patients fail."

- Worsening renal function and outcome [14]
  Among elderly patients with CHF, those whose creatinine increased ≥ 0.5 mg/dL within the first 6 months on HF treatment had nearly ×2 higher mortality rate compared with those who didn't have worsening of creatinine.

CKD class and outcome [15].

- Nearly 55% of HF pts. have eGFR<60

Fig. 28.2 CKD stage affect survival

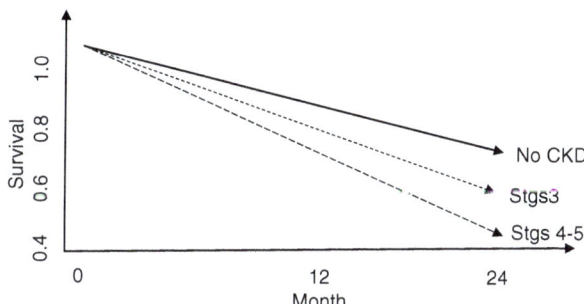

Table 28.7 "# of HF admissions directly affect the survival"

Medial survival (years) after HF admissions	
# of admission	Medial survival (years)
1	2.4
2	1.4
3	1.0
4	0.6

Setoguchi et al. [16]

References

1. ☺ ☺ ☺Cotter G, et al. The pathophysiology of acute heart failure-Is it all about fluid accumulation? Am Heart J. 2008;155:9–18.
2. Kittleson M, Kobashigawa J. Management of advanced heart failure. The role of heart transplantation. Circulation. 2011;123:1569–74.
3. ☺ ☺Kapoor J, Perazellas M. Diagnostic and therapeutic approach to acute decompensated heart failure. Am J Med. 2007;120:121–7.
4. ☺Stevenson L. Tailored therapy to hemodynamic goals for advanced heart failure. Eur J Heart Failure. 1999;1:251–7.
5. ☺ ☺ ☺Hollenberg S, et al. 2019 ACC expert consensus decision pathway on risk assessment, management, and clinical trajectory of patients hospitalized with heart failure. J Am Coll Cardiol. 2019;74:1966–2011.
6. Gilstrap L, et al. Reasons for guideline nonadherence at heart failure discharge. J Am Heart Assoc. 2018;7:e008789. https://doi.org/10.1161/JAHA.118.008789.
7. ☺ ☺Ricci Z, et al. Cardiorenal syndrome. Crit Care Clin. 2021;37:335–47.

8. Jentzer J, et al. Contemporary management of severe acute kidney injury and refractory cardiorenal syndrome. J Am Coll Cardiol. 2020;76:1084–101.

9. Ambrosy A, et al. Clinical course and predictive value of congestion during hospitalization in patients admitted for worsening signs and symptoms of HFrEF findings from the EVEREST trial. Eur Heart J. 2013;34:835–43.

10. Lewis E, et al. The association of the heart failure score with mortality and heart failure hospitalizations in elderly patients: insights from the Mode Selection Trial (MOST). Am Heart J. 2006;151:699–705.

11. Chioncel O, et al. Acute heart failure congestion and perfusion status – impact of the clinical classification on in-hospital and long-term outcomes; insights from the ESC-EORP-HFA Heart Failure Long-Term Registry. Eur J Heart Failure. 2019;21:1338–52.

12. Fonarow G, et al. Risk stratification for in-hospital mortality in acutely decompensated heart failure. Classification and regression tree analysis. JAMA. 2005;293:572–80.

13. Lee D, et al. Prediction of heart failure mortality in emergent care. Ann Intern Med. 2012;156:767–75.

14. Maeder M, et al. Incidence, clinical predictors, and prognostic impact of worsening renal funcion in elderly patients with chronic heart failure on intensive medical therapy. Am Heart J. 2012;163:407–414.e401.

15. ☺ ☺ House A. Management of heart failure in advancing CKD: Core curriculum 2018. Am J Kidney Dis. 2018;72(2):284–95.

16. Setoguchi S, et al. Repeated hospitalizations predict mortality in the community population with heart failure. Am Heart J. 2007;154:260–6.

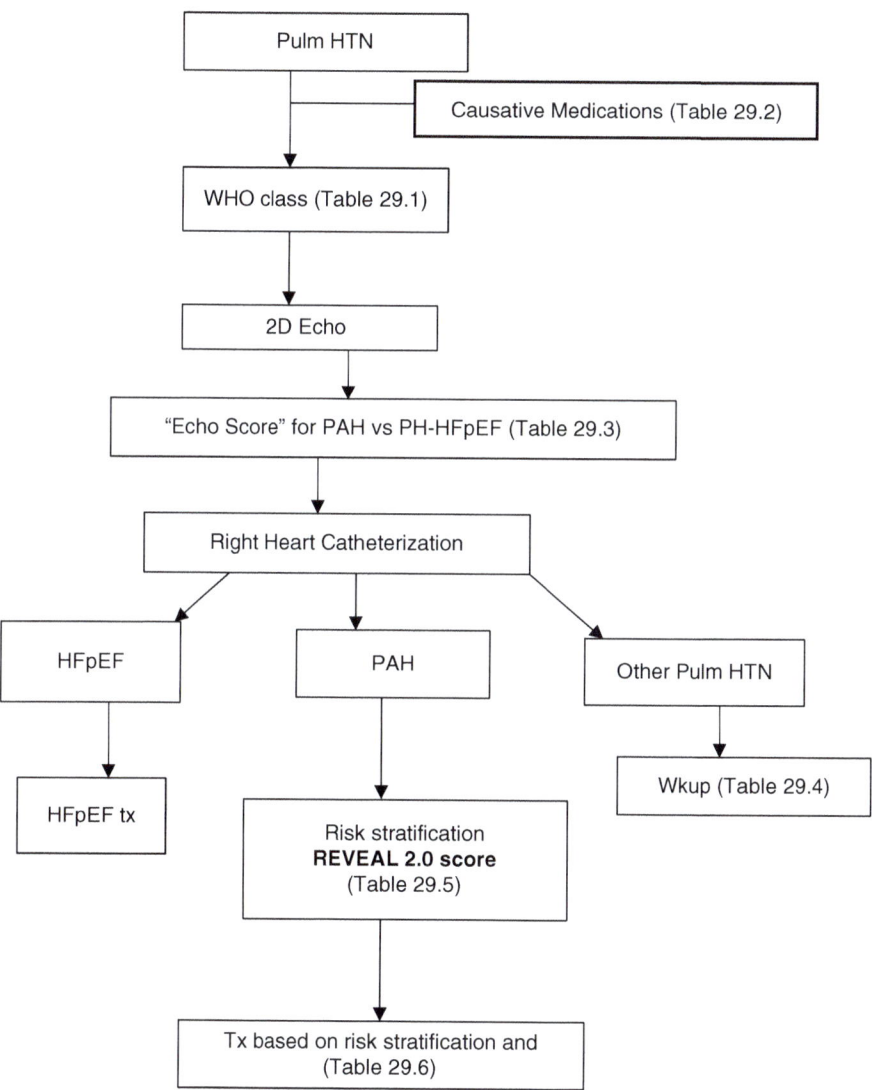

Fig. 29.1 Overview

M. J. Morikawa, *The Inpatient Medicine Handbook*,
https://doi.org/10.1007/978-3-032-08398-2_29

Definition:

New definition mPAP > 20 mmHg [1]

Table 29.1 Classification

• Two classifications: (1) based on etiology and (2) based on hemodynamics		
Hemodynamic based	WHO class	Examples
Precapillary Increased PA resistance PAP > 20 mmHg PAWP ≤ 15 mmHg PVR ≥ 3 WU	Arterial HTN	Idiopathic, heritable, toxin/drug induced, connective tissue disease HIV infection
Postcapillary Increased resistance distal to pulmonary capillaries PAP > 20 mmHg PAWP > 15 mmHg PVR ≥ 3 WU combined pre- + postcapillary Or PVR < 3 WU if isolated postcapillary	Left heart disease	HFpEF, HFrEF, valvular HD
	Lung disease/ hypoxia	COPD, restrictive lung disease, obesity-hypoventilation, developmental lung disease
	PA obstruction	Chronic PE
	Idiopathic	Hematological disorders, SCD, sarcoidosis

Maron et al. [2]; Ruopp and Cockrill [1]; Hassoun [3]

Hemodynamic categorization

PAP > 20 mmHg		
PAWP ≤ 15	PAWP > 15	
PVR ≥ 3 WU	PVR ≥ 3 WU	PVR < 3 WU
Precapillary PH	Combined pre- + postcapillary PH	Isolated postcapillary PH

Galie et al. [4]; Maron et al. [2]

Table 29.2 Medications causing Pulm HTN

Definite	Likely	Possible
Aminorex Fenfluramine SSRI	Amphetamines Methamphetamines	Cocaine St John's wort Interferon α and β Alkylating agents

Galie et al. [4]; Maron et al. [2]

Table 29.3 Echocardiogram score to differentiate PAH vs PH-HFpEF score ≥ 0 PPV 68% for PAH

Variable	Point
E/e′ > 10	−1
LA AP dimension >4.2 cm	−1
LA AP dimension <3.2 cm	+1
RVOT PW Doppler midsystolic notch or AccT < 80 ms	+1

Opotowsky et al. [5]

Table 29.4 Workup

Imaging:
High resolution chest CT
V/Q scan
Blood
BNP, NT-proBNP, ANA, LFTs, hepatitis, HIV
PFT

Hassoun [3]

Table 29.5 REVEAL risk score (2.0)

Variable	Points
WHO group I subgroup	
Connective tissue disease	1
Portopulmonary HTN	3
Familial PAH	2
Demographics & comorbidities	
Renal insufficiency eGFR < 60	1
Male age > 60	2
NYHA/WHO functional class	
I	−1
III	1
IV	2
Vital signs	
SBP < 110 mmHg	1
HR > 92	1
6-min walk	
≥440 m	−2
320 to <440 m	−1
<165 m	1
BNP	
<50 pg/mL or NT-proBNP < 300 pg/mL	−2
BNP 200 to <800	1
BNP ≥ 800 or NT-proBNP ≥ 1100 pg/mL	2
Echocardiogram	
Pericardial effusion	1
PFT	
% pred.DLco < 40	1
Right heart catheterization	
mRAP > 20 mmHg within 1 year	1
PVR < 5 Wood units	−1

Benza et al. [6, 7]

$$REVEAL \text{ risk score} = \text{sum of above} + 6$$

Risk category and score with 1-year survival (REVEAL original score)

Risk category	Score	1-Year survival (%)
Low	1–7	95.2
Average	8	91.5
Moderate	9	88.6
High	10–11	71.9
Very high	≥12	65.9

Risk stratification based on REVEAL

Risk category	REVEAL score
Low	0–6
Intermediate	7–8
High	≥9

2022 ESC/ERS risk stratification introduced three-strata and four-strata model for risk assessment [8]

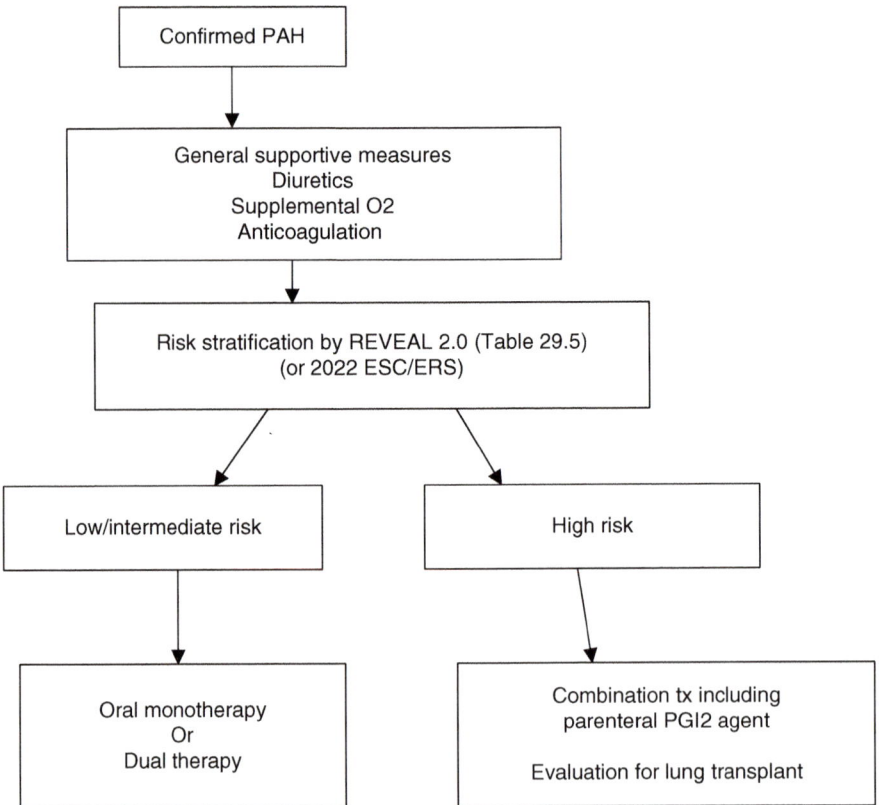

Fig. 29.2 Treatment strategies [3]

Table 29.6 Treatment

Three pathways of targeted therapy in PAH	
Pathway	Medication
Endothelin-1 pathway	Ambrisentan
	Bosentan
	Macitentan
Prostacyclin (PGI2) pathway	Epoprostenol
	Treprostinil
	Iloprost
	Selexipag
Nitric oxide pathway	Riociguat
	Sildenafil
	Tadalafil

Hassoun [3]

References

1. Ruopp N, Cockrill B. Diagnosis and treatment of pulmonary arterial hypertension. A review. JAMA. 2022;327(14):1379–91.
2. Maron B, et al. Pulmonary arterial hypertension: diagnosis, treatment, and novel advances. Am J Respir Crit Care Med. 2021;203(12):1472–87.
3. ☺Hassoun P. Pulmonary arterial hypertension. N Engl J Med. 2021;385:2361–76.
4. Galie N, et al. 2015 ESC/ERS guidelines for the diagnosis and treatment of pulmonary hypertension. Eur Respir J. 2015;46:903–75.
5. Opotowsky A, et al. A simple echocardiographic prediction rule for hemodynamics in pulmonary hypertension. Circ Cardiovasc Imaging. 2012;5:765–75.
6. Benza R, et al. The REVEAL registry risk score calculator in patients newly diagnosed with pulmonary arterial hypertension. Chest. 2012;141(2):354–62.
7. ☺☺Benza R, et al. Predicting survival in patients with pulmonary arterial hypertension. The REVEAL risk score calculator 2.0 and comparison with ESC/ERS-based risk assessment strategies. Chest. 2019;156:323–37.
8. ☺☺Humbert M, et al. 2022 ESC/ERS guidelines for the diagnosis and treatment of pulmonary hypertension. Eur Heart J. 2022;43:3618–731.

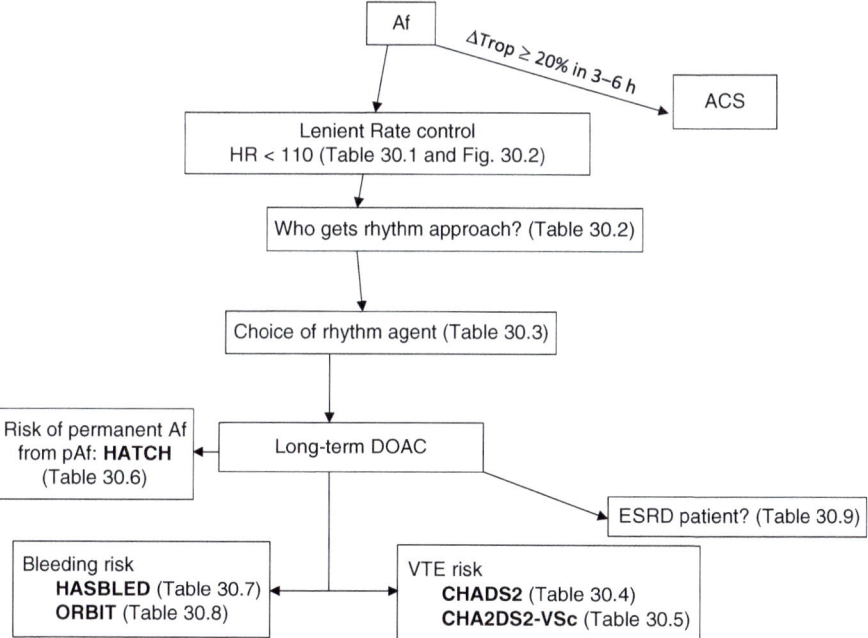

Fig. 30.1 Big picture

© The Author(s), under exclusive license to Springer Nature Switzerland AG 2025
M. J. Morikawa, *The Inpatient Medicine Handbook*,
https://doi.org/10.1007/978-3-032-08398-2_30

Facts:

- Lifetime risk of Af above 40 y/o is approx. 25% [1]
- Af risk above 55 y/o is 37% [2]
- Paroxysmal Af develops to persistent AF 5–10%/year [2]

RFs:

- Age, male, obesity, T2DM, dyslipidemia, HTN, OSA, EToH [3]
- Strong correlation between length of tx for DM and Af risk [4]

Path:

- Three factors: Structural remodeling, electrical remodeling and inflammation [5]
- The most common ectopic atrial beats that triggers Af are in myocardial sleeves [1, 6]

Definitions [7]

Paroxysmal (lasting <7 days)
Persistent (>7 days)
Permanent (>1 year or refractory to cardioversion)

Diagnosis:

Chest pain in Af due to RVR vs ACS [8]

- Troponin change >40% or absolute change of 50 ng/dL in hs-cTnI = type 1 MI
- >20% change from the baseline is suspicious for type 1 MI

MGMT:

Big picture:
1. Rate control
2. Stroke prevention (anticoagulation or procedure)
3. Upstream intervention or risk MGMT [4]
4. Long-term strategy (rhythm vs rate control)

Michaud and Stevenson [2]

Rate control approach [9]

- Lenient rate control: HR <110 (Van Gelder NEJ [10])
- Consider rhythm control or AV nodal ablation if worsening LV function or tachy-cardiomyopathy persist or continuous bi-V pacing in CRT is not achieved.

Fig. 30.2 Acute rate control in Af with RVR

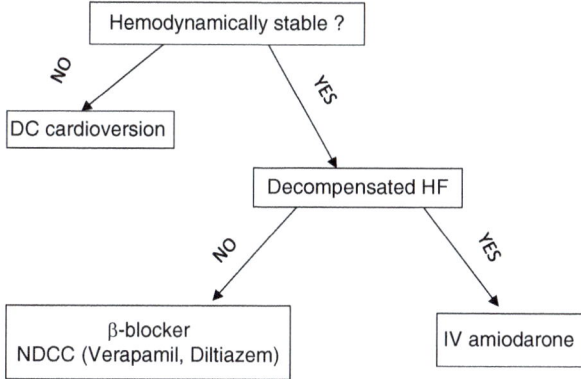

Table 30.1 Long-term rate control

	EF ≤ 40%	EF > 40%
First choice	β-Blocker	β-Blocker or NDCC
Second choice	Digoxin	Digoxin

Van Gelder et al. [9]; Joglar et al. [11]

Stroke prevention: DOAC

- The risk of stroke is highest in the first 72 h after cardioversion [12]
- Oral anticoagulation should be continued for at least 2–3 months after ablation and thereafter should be on the basis of patients' underlying risk score (CHADSVASc >1 for men, >2 for women) rather than the rhythm status [12]

Table 30.2 Who gets rhythm control?

LV dysfunction
Moderate or severe symptoms from Af
Age < 80 y/o
Worsening symptoms or cardiac function with rate control
       Elderly (age > 80), frail = RATE CONTROL

Joglar et al. [11]; Wiggins et al. [13]; Van Gelder et al. [9]

Table 30.3 Rhythm control medications and modalities

	Normal LV EF, no SHD	HFrEF or SHD
First choice	Dofetilide	Amiodarone
	Dronedarone	Dofetilide
	Flecainide	
	Propafenone	
Second choice	Amiodarone	Sotalol

Joglar et al. [11]; Piccini and Fauchier [12]; Prystowsky et al. [14]

- Ablation is most successful in paroxysmal Af with no structural HD [15]
- Recurrence rate after ablation 6–9%/year [16]
- Recommends Holter Q3–6 months for 2 years after ablation
- New risk stratification for CVA in Af by D-dimer and vWf? [17]

Prognosis:

- Prediction of development of Af (CHADS2, CHA2DS2-VSc, CHARGE-AF)

Table 30.4 CHADS2 score

Variable and point	
Variable	Point
CHF	1
HTN (>140/90)	1
Age ≥75	1
DM	1
TIA or stroke	2
CHADS2 score and event rate in 1-year	
Score	Event rate (%)
0	1.67
1	4.75
2	7.34
3	15.47
4	21.55
5	19.71
6	22.36
Risk category and event rate in 1 year	
Risk category	Event rate (%)
Low risk (0)	1.67
Intermediate (1)	4.75
High (2–6)	12.27

Table 30.5 CHADSVASc score

Variable and point	
Variable	Point
CHF	1
HTN (>140/90)	1
Age ≥75	2
DM	1
TIA or stroke	2
Vascular disease (MI, aortic plague etc)	1
Age 65–74	1
Female	1

Chung et al. [18]

CHADSVASc score and event rate at 1-year		
Score	Event rate (%)	Event rate in original NICE cohort
0	0.78	0
1	2.01	0.6
2	3.71	1.6
3	5.92	3.9
4	9.27	1.9
5	15.26	3.2
6	19.74	3.6
7	21.50	8.0
8	22.38	11.0
9	23.64	100
Risk category and event rate		
Risk category	Event rate (%)	
Low risk (0)	0.78	
Intermediate (1)	2.01	
High risk (2–9)	8.82	

Olesen et al. [19]; Lip et al. [20]

- CHADSVASc ≥2 should be on anticoagulation [2]
- Both CHADS2 ≥2 and CHADSVASc ≥3 are predictor of developing new onset Af

Table 30.6 HATCH score

- Progression from paroxysmal Af to persistent Af [18, 21]	
- HATCH score ≥2 also predict new-onset Af after catheter ablation of Aflutter [22]	
Variable and point	
Variable	Point
HTN	1
Age ≥75	1
TIA or stroke	2
COPD	1
HF	2
HATCH score and incidence of persistent Af in 10 years	
Score	Incidence
0	0.8
1	7.3
2	9.9
3	10.5
4	18.0
5	20.5
6	32.3
7	57.3

Suenari et al. [23]

Long-term anticoagulation [24]
- Bleeding risk assessment

Table 30.7 HASBLED score

	Variable	Point
H	HTN	1
A	Abnormal renal function	1
	Abnormal liver function	1
S	Stroke	1
B	Bleeding	1
L	Labile INRs	1
E	Elderly (>65)	1
D	Drugs	1
	Alcohol	1

Pisters et al. [25]

- HAS-BLED low (score 0–1) 2.54%, intermediate (score 2) 5.4%, and high (score ≥3) 7.68% [26]

Event rate based on HASBLED score

Score	Event rate (%)
0	1.13
1	1.02
2	1.88
3	3.74
4	8.7
5	12.5
≥6	Too rare

Table 30.8 ORBIT score

- ORBIT provides the most accurate level of absolute bleeding risk https://www.mdcalc.com/orbt-bleeding-risk-score-atrial-fibrillation

	Variable	Point
O	Older (≥75)	1
R	Reduced hemoglobin Men <13 mg/dL, Ht < 40% Women <12 mg/dL, Ht < 36%	2
B	Bleeding history GI bleeding, intracranial bleeding or hemorrhagic stroke	2
I	Insufficient kidney function (eGFR <60 mg/dL/1.73 m)	1
T	Treatment with antiplatelet	1

Event rate by scores	
ORBIT score	Major bleeding rate (%)
0	1.7
1	2.3
2	2.9
3	4.7
4	6.8
5	9.0
6	12.3
7	14.9

O'Brien (2015); Perry et al. [27]

Table 30.9 Advanced renal disease patients with Af

CKD stage	eGFR	Modalities
1	≥90	DOAC
2	60–89	
3a	45–59	
3b	30–44	
4	15–29	No RCT for anticoagulation available
5	<15	Non-pharmacologic tx or no tx
5D	–	If treat, DOAC preferred over VKA

FDA guide for dosing					
CKD stage	eGFR	Dabigatran	Apixaban	Rivaroxaban	Edoxaban
4	15–30	75 mg BID	5/2.5 mg BID	15 mg QD	30 mg QD
5	<15	–	5 mg BID	–	–
5D	HD	–	5 mg BID	–	–

Kumar et al. [28]

References

1. Morin D, et al. The state of the art: atrial fibrillation epidemiology, prevention, and treatment. Mayo Clin Proc. 2016;91(12):1778–810.
2. ☺☺Michaud G, Stevenson W. Atrial fibrillation. N Engl J Med. 2021;384:353–61.
3. Menezes A, et al. Atrial fibrillation in the 21st century: a current understanding of risk factors and primary prevention strategies. Mayo Clin Proc. 2013;88(4):394–409.

4. Wang A, et al. Atrial fibrillation and diabetes mellitus. J Am Coll Cardiol. 2019;74:1107–15.
5. Kourliouros A, et al. Current opinion in the pathogenesis of atrial fibrillation. Am Heart J. 2009;157:243–52.
6. Lubitz S, et al. Catheter ablation for atrial fibrillation. BMJ. 2008;336:819–26.
7. Eagle K, et al. Management of atrial fibrillation: translating clinical trial data into clinical practice. Am J Med. 2011;124:4–14.
8. ☺☺Chang K, et al. Clinical applications of biomarkers in atrial fibrillation. Am J Med. 2017;130:1351–7.
9. ☺☺☺van Gelder I, et al. Atrial fibrillation 2. Rate control in atrial fibrillation. Lancet. 2016;388:818–28.
10. Van Gelder I, et al. Lenient versus strict rate control in patients with atrial fibrillation. N Engl J Med. 2010;362:1363–73.
11. ☺☺☺Joglar J, et al. 2023 ACC/AHA/ACCP/HRS guideline for the diagnosis and management of atrial fibrillation: a report of the American College of Cardiology/American Heart Association Joint Committee on clinical practice guidelines. Circulation. 2024;149:e1–e156. https://doi.org/10.1161/CIR0000000000001193.
12. ☺☺Piccini J, Fauchier L. Atrial fibrillation 3. Rhythm control in atrial fibrillation. Lancet. 2016;388:829–40.
13. Wiggins B, et al. 2023 Atrial fibrillation guideline-at-a-glance. J Am Coll Cardiol. 2024;83(1):280–4.
14. ☺☺Prystowsky E, et al. Treatment of atrial fibrillation. JAMA. 2015;314(3):278–88.
15. Link M, et al. Ablation of atrial fibrillation. Circulation. 2016;134:339–52.
16. Wazni O, et al. Catheter ablation for atrial fibrillation. N Engl J Med. 2011;365:2296–304.
17. Watson T, et al. Mechanisms of thrombogenesis in atrial fibrillation: Virchow's triad revisited. Lancet. 2009;373:155–66.
18. Chung M, et al. Atrial fibrillation. J Am Coll Cardiol. 2020;75:1689–713.
19. Olesen J, et al. Validation of risk stratification schemes for predicting stroke and thromboembolism in patients with atrial fibrillation: nationwide cohort study. BMJ. 2011;342:d124. https://doi.org/10.1136/bmj.d124.
20. Lip G, et al. Refining clinical risk stratification for predicting stroke and thromboembolism in atrial fibrillation using a novel risk factor-based approach. Chest. 2010;137(2):263–72.
21. de Vos C, et al. Progression from paroxysmal to persistent atrial fibrillation. J Am Coll Cardiol. 2010;55:725–31.
22. Chen K, et al. HATCH score in the prediction of new-onset atrial fibrillation after catheter ablation of typical atrial flutter. Heart Rhythm. 2015;12:1483–9.
23. Suenari K, et al. Usefulness of HATCH score in the prediction of new-onset atrial fibrillation for Asians. Medicine (Baltimore). 2017;96:e5597. https://doi.org/10.1097/MD.0000000000005597.
24. Lip G, et al. Antithrombotic therapy for atrial fibrillation. CHEST guideline and expert panel report. Chest. 2018;154(5):1121–201.
25. Pisters R, et al. A novel user-friendly score (HAS-BLED) to assess 1-year risk of major bleeding in patients with atrial fibrillation. The Euro Heart Study. Chest. 2010;138:1093–100.
26. ☺☺Olesen J, et al. Bleeding risk in 'real world' patients with atrial fibrillation: comparison of two established bleeding prediction schemes in a nationwide cohort. J Thromb Haemost. 2011;9:1460–7.
27. Perry M, et al. Atrial fibrillation: diagnosis and management-summary of NICE guidance. BMJ. 2021;373:n1150. https://doi.org/10.1136/bmj.n1150.
28. ☺Kumar S, et al. Anticoagulation in concomitant chronic kidney disease and atrial fibrillation. J Am Coll Cardiol. 2019;74:2204–15.

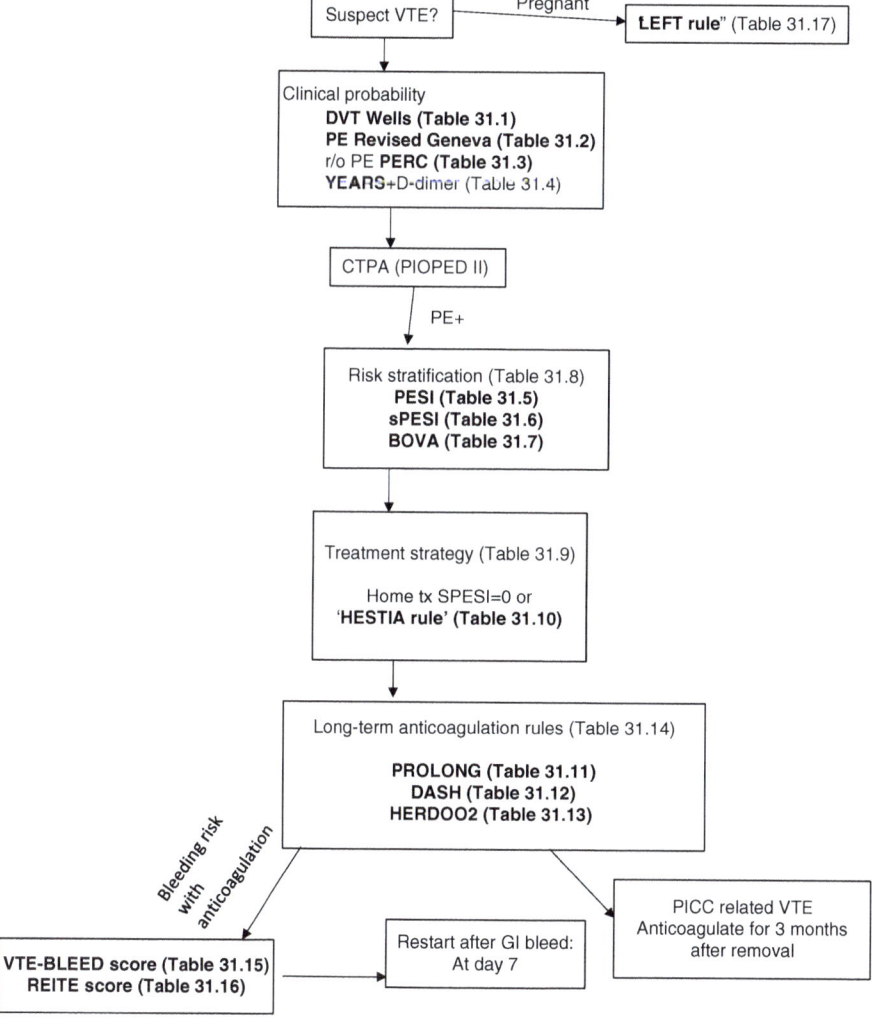

Fig. 31.1 Big picture

© The Author(s), under exclusive license to Springer Nature Switzerland AG 2025

M. J. Morikawa, *The Inpatient Medicine Handbook*,

https://doi.org/10.1007/978-3-032-08398-2_31

- First unprovoked VTE has a high risk of recurrence 10% after 1 year and 30% at 5 years [1]
- Recurrence rate of VTE was similar if stopped at 3 months compared with 6 months or later.
- Recurrence rate was higher during the first 6 months after stopping the anticoagulation [2]

Clinical Risk Stratification

Dx algorithm for PE

PIOPED II [3]

Table 31.1 Wells score

Variable	Points
PE is the most likely Dx	3
Signs and symptoms of DVT	3
HR > 100	1.5
Immobilization >3 days or surgery <4 weeks	1.5
Previous VTE	1.5
Hemoptysis	1
Active cancer	1

Score ≤ 4 low clinical probability

Table 31.2 PE: Revised Geneva

Variable	Points
Age ≥ 65	1
Previous VTE	3
Surgery or fx < 1 month	2
Active malignancy	2
Unilateral lower limb pain	3
Hemoptysis	2
HR 75–94	3
HR ≥ 95	5
Pain on palpation on lower limb and unilateral edema	4

Score ≤ 10 is low probability

- D-dimer cut-off: (patient's age × 10) µg/L in patients aged > 50 [4]

R/O PE

Table 31.3 PERC rule

• If all the answer is no, PE risk is low

1. Age > 49
2. HR > 99
3. Pox < 95% (RA)
4. Hx of hemoptysis
5. On estrogen
6. Hx of VTE
7. Recent surgery or trauma
8. Unilateral leg swelling

Kline et al. [5]

Table 31.4 YEARS rule

D-dimer + 3 YEARS questions:
  Clinical signs of DVT
  Hemoptysis
  PE is the most likely Dx

Procedures:

0 YEARS items + D dimer <1000 ng/mL	PE ruled out
0 YEARS items + D-dimer ≥1000	Order CTPA
≥1 YEARS items + D-dimer <500	PE ruled out
≥1 YEARS items + D-dimer ≥500	Order CTPA

Van der Hulle et al. [6]

Diagnosis based on rules and scans [7]
PE is r/o when

PERC negative
No YEARS + D-dimer <1000
≥1 YEARS + D-dimer <500
Wells score ≤4 + D-dimer <1000
Revised Geneva ≤10 + D-dimer <1000 ng/mL

Risk stratification:
RV strain:

- A value of <1.0 for the ratio of the RV diameter to the LV diameter had a 100% negative predictive value for an uneventful outcome [8]
- 2DEcho evidence of spectrum of RV strain [9]

Submassive or intermediate risk patients

Table 31.5 PESI score

Variable	Points
Demographics	
Age (years)	Age
Male	10
Comorbidity	
Cancer	30
HF	10
Chronic lung disease	10
Clinical findings	
Pulse ≥ 110	20
SBP < 100	30
RR ≥ 30	20
Temp < 36 °C	20
Altered mental status	60
Pox < 90%	20

Class	Score	Mortality (%)
I	<65	0
II	66–85	1.0
III	86–105	3.1
IV	106–125	12.9
V	125<	24.4

Aujesky et al. [10]

Table 31.6 sPESI score

Variable	Points
Age > 80	1
Hx of cancer	1
Hx of chronic cardiopulmonary disease	1
Pulse ≥ 110	1
SBPM < 100 mmHg	1
Pox < 90%	1

Risk category and mortality		
Risk category	Points	Morality (%)
Low	0	2.5
High	≥1	10.9

Stamm [11]; Jimenez et al. [12]

Table 31.7 BOVA score: SBP, Tp, RV dysfunction on CT, HR >110

Variable	Points
SBP 90–100 mmHg	2
Elevated troponin	2
RV dysfunction on Echo or CT	2
HR ≥ 110	1

Stage	Points	30-day PE related mortality (%)
I	0–2	1.7
II	3–4	5.0
III	4<	15.5

Bova et al. [13]

Table 31.8 PE Risk stratification biomarker, PESI, sPESI, RV strain

Mortality risk	Hemodynamic instability	PESI III–V or sPESI ≥ 1	RV strain on imaging	Troponin
High	+	+	+	+
Intermediate-high	–	+	Both positive	
Intermediate-low	–	+	Either or none positive	
Low	–	–	–	–

Konstantinides et al. [14]; Piazza [9]

Table 31.9 Treatment strategy

Low	Intermediate		High
sPESI = 0	sPESI ≥ 1 and SBP ≥ 90		Hemodynamically unstable
HESTIA = 0	Intermediate-low	Intermediate-high	
	NoRVstrainorTrop-	RV strain + Trop +	
Home/ DOAC	Admit/DOAC	Admit heparin, start DOAC <72 h	MICU/thrombolysis

Piazza [9]; Freund [33]

Home treatment or not [7, 15, 16]

$$\text{Hestia}: \text{all no or sPESI} = 0 : \text{home treatment}\,[7]$$

Table 31.10 Hestia rule

• All answers are no, then home tx
Hemodynamically unstable
Thrombolysis/embolectomy necessary
Active bleeding or high risk for bleed
Oxygen >24 h to maintain Pox > 90%
PE while on anticoagulation
Severe pain needing IV pain med > 24 h
Medical/social reason for tx in inpatient > 24 h
Creatinine clearance < 30 mL/min
Have severe liver impairment
Pregnant
Hx of HIT

Zondag et al. [16]

Prediction for Recurrence

- Recurrence risk of VTE: approximately 25% at 4 years and first 2 years are the highest.
- Annual recurrence rate approximately 10% in each of the first 2 years [17]
- Highest rate of recurrence was within 6 months after stopping anticoagulation [2]

Table 31.11 PROLONG protocol

• D-dimer 1 months after the discontinuation of anticoagulation

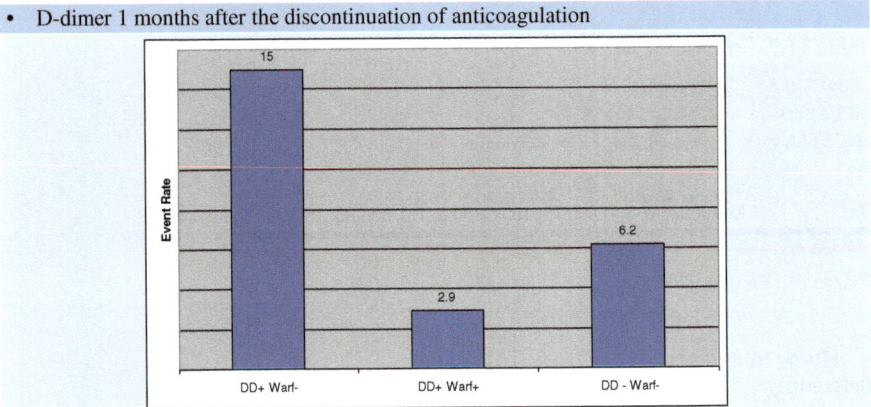

Palareti et al. [18]

Table 31.12 DASH score

Variable	Points
D-dimer abnormal 30 days after stopping anticoagulation	2
Age ≤ 50	1
Male	1
Hormone-use proved VTE	−2

Risk stratification and procedure		
Score	Annual recurrence rate (%)	Decision
≤1	3.1	STOP anticoagulation
2	6.4	Continue
3≤	12.3	Continue

Tosetto et al. [19]

Table 31.13 HERDOO2

Variable	Point

Post-thrombotic signs
  Hyperpigmentation
  Edema
  Redness
	1 point for any of these signs

D-dimer ≥ 250 µg/L	1
BMI ≥ 30	1
Age ≥ 65	1

Decision-making		
Women		Men
0–1	≥2	Continue
Discontinue	Continue	

Rodger et al. [20]

Anticoagulation

Table 31.14 Length of tx

After finishing 3–6 months of anticoagulation:					
	Isolated distal DVT or subsegmental PE	Provoked VTE (Including catheter associated)	First unproved VTE		Active cancer APL Ab ≥2 unprovoked VTE
			Women with HERDOO2 ≤ 1	Women with HERDOO2 ≥ 2 + All men	
Major bleeding risk +					
STOP anticoagulation				CONTINUE anticoagulation	

Khan et al. [21]; Renner and Barnes [22]

Thrombophilia workup?

- More than 50% of initial episode of VTE is idiopathic.
- The rate of recurrence in patients with thrombophilia (2.5%) was the same as the total group (2.6%), but the rate of recurrence in patient in idiopathic was higher (3.3%).

Patients with an initial VTE, the risk of recurrent VTE is greater if the episode was idiopathic than if it occurred with thrombophilia.

Dalen [23]

Who should be tested?

Thrombosis <50 y/o with weak provoking factor
Strong family hx of VTE
Recurrent VTE at young age
VTE in unusual site: splanchnic or cerebral veins

Connors [24]

Bleeding Risk Score

Table 31.15 VTE-BLEED score

Variable	Points
• Score ≥2 high risk	
Active cancer	2
Male with uncontrolled HTN	1
Anemia	1.5
Hx of bleeding	1.5
CKD (CCr 30–60)	1.5
Age ≥ 60	1.5

Klok and Huisman [25]

Table 31.16 REITE score

Variable	Points
Recent major bleed	2
Creatinine >1.2 mg/dL	1.5
Hb < 13 g/dL (male) or 12 g/dL (female)	1.5
Malignancy	1
Clinically overt PE	1
Age > 75	1

Risk of bleeding	
Score	Probability (%)
0	0.3
1–4	2.6
4<	7.3

Goldhaber and Bounameaux [26]; Ruiz-Gimenez et al. [27]

After GI Bleeding…

• Resume anticoagulation for VTE after 7 days but within 15 days
(restarting after 7 days was not associated with increased risk of GIB but was associated with decreased risk of mortality and VTE compared with resuming after 30 days [28].

PICC Related VTE

• DVT+ and PICC is NOT needed anymore, anticoagulated with UFH or LMWH for 3–5 days then remove. Anticoagulation for 3 months after the removal.
• If DVT + and PICC is NEEDED, anticoagulated LMWH for 3–6 months [29]

Pregnancy

Table 31.17 LEFT rule

If none of three variables
Left side symptoms
Circumference difference ≥ 2 cm
Or first trimester
Then DVT unlikely.

Chan et al. [30]

Prophylaxis

• CAPRINI score [31]
• Trauma patient [32]

TBI pt use Modified Berne   Norwood criteria

References

1. ☺ ☺ ☺ Tritschler T, et al. Venous thromboembolism. Advances in diagnosis and treatment. JAMA. 2018;320(15):1583–94.
2. Boutitie F, et al. Influence of preceding length of anticoagulant treatment and initial presentation of venous thromboembolism on risk of recurrence after stopping treatment: analysis of individual participants' data from seven trials. BMJ. 2011;342:d3036. https://doi.org/10.1136/bmj.d3036.
3. Stein P, et al. Diagnosis pathways in acute pulmonary embolism: recommendations of the PIOPED II investigators. Am J Med. 2006;119:1048–55.
4. Douma R, et al. Potential of an age adjusted D-dimer cut-off value to improve the exclusion of pulmonary embolism in older patients: a retrospective analysis of three large cohorts. BMJ. 2010;340:c1475. https://doi.org/10.1136/bmj.c1475.
5. Kline J, et al. Prospective multicenter evaluation of the pulmonary embolism rule-out criteria. J Thromb Haemost. 2008;6:772–80.
6. van der Hulle T, et al. Simplified diagnostic management of suspected pulmonary embolism (the YEARS study): a prospective, multicenter, cohort study. Lancet. 2017;390:289–97.

7. ☺☺☺Kahn S, de Wit K. Pulmonary embolism. N Engl J Med. 2022;387:45–57.
8. Agnelli G, Becattini C. Acute pulmonary embolism. N Engl J Med. 2010;363:266–74.
9. ☺☺Piazza G. Advanced management of intermediate- and high-risk pulmonary embolism. J Am Coll Cardiol. 2020;76:2117–27.
10. Aujesky D, et al. Validation of a model to predict adverse outcomes in patients with pulmonary embolism. Eur Heart J. 2006;27:476–81.
11. ☺Stamm J. Risk stratification for acute pulmonary embolism. Crit Care Clin. 2012;28:301–21.
12. Jimenez D, et al. Simplification of the Pulmonary Embolism Severity Index for prognostication in patients with acute symptomatic pulmonary embolism. Arch Intern Med. 2010;170(15):1383–9.
13. Bova C, et al. Identification of intermediate-risk patients with acute symptomatic pulmonary embolism. Eur Respir J. 2014;44:694–703.
14. Konstantinides S, et al. Management of pulmonary embolism. J Am Coll Cardiol. 2016;67:976–90.
15. Roy P, et al. Triaging acute pulmonary embolism for home treatment by Hestia or simplified PESI criteria: the HOME-PE randomized trial. Eur Heart J. 2021;42:3146–57.
16. Zondag W, et al. Outpatient treatment in patients with acute pulmonary embolism: the Hestia study. J Thromb Haemost. 2011;9:1500–7.
17. Bauer K. Long-term management of venous thromboembolism. A 61-year-old woman with unprovoked venous thromboembolism. JAMA. 2011;305:1336–45.
18. ☺Palareti G, et al. D-dimer testing to determine the duration of anticoagulation therapy. N Engl J Med. 2006;355:1780–9.
19. Tosetto A, et al. Predicting disease recurrence in patients with previous unprovoked venous thromboembolism: a proposed prediction score (DASH). J Thromb Haemost. 2012;10:1019–25.
20. Rodger M, et al. Identifying unprovoked thromboembolism patients at low risk for recurrence who can discontinue anticoagulant therapy. CMAJ. 2008;179(5):417–26.
21. Khan F, et al. Venous thromboembolism. Lancet. 2021;398:64–77.
22. ☺☺☺Renner E, Barnes G. Antithrombotic management of venous thromboembolism. J Am Coll Cardiol. 2020;76:2142–54.
23. Dalen J. Should patients with venous thromboembolism be screened for thrombophilia? Am J Med. 2008;121:458–63.
24. ☺☺☺Connors J. Thrombophilia testing and venous thrombosis. N Engl J Med. 2017;377:1177–87.
25. Klok F, Huisman M. How I assess and manage the risk of bleeding in patients treated for venous thromboembolism. Blood. 2020;135(10):724–34.
26. Goldhaber S, Bounameaux H. Pulmonary embolism and deep vein thrombosis. Lancet. 2012;379:1835–46.
27. Ruiz-Gimenez N, et al. Predictive variables for major bleeding events in patients presenting with documented acute venous thromboembolism. Findings from the RIETE registry. Thromb Haemost. 2008;100:26–31.
28. ☺Qureshi W, et al. Restarting anticoagulation and outcomes after major gastrointestinal bleeding in atrial fibrillation. Am J Cardiol. 2014;113:662–8.
29. Baskin J, et al. Management of occlusion and thrombosis associated with long-term indwelling central venous catheters. Lancet. 2009;374:159–69.
30. Chan W, et al. Predicting deep vein thrombosis in pregnancy: out in "LEFt" field? Ann Intern Med. 2009;151:85–92.
31. Gould M, et al. Prevention of VTE in nonorthopedic surgical patients. Chest. 2012;141(2 suppl):e227S–77S.
32. Yorkgitis B, et al. American Association for the Surgery of Trauma/American College of Surgeons-Committee on Trauma Clinical Protocol for inpatient venous thromboembolism prophylaxis after trauma. J Trauma Acute Care Surg. 2022;92(3):597–604.
33. Freund Y, Cohen-Aubart F, Bloom B. "Acute pulmonary embolism. A review" JAMA 2022;328:1336–45.

Pneumonia

32

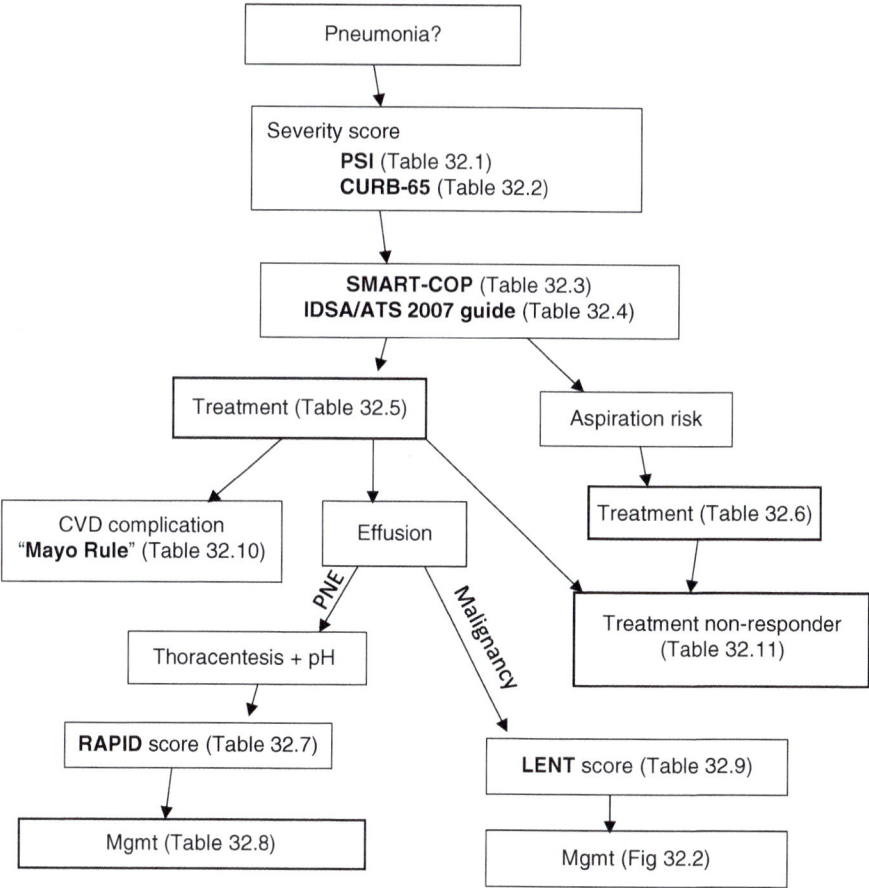

Fig. 32.1 Workflow

FACTS:

• 1/3 of patients dying within 1 year after discharge from hospital for pneumonia [1]

Severity Score:

Table 32.1 PSI (Pneumonia Severity Index)

Variable	Points
Age	
Men	Age (year)
Women	Age (year) −10
Nursing home resident	10
Coexisting illnesses	
Cancer	30
Liver disease	20
CHF	10
CVA	10
Renal disease	10
PE findings	
Altered mental status	20
RR ≥ 30	20
SBP < 90 mmHg	20
Temperature <35 or ≥40 °C	15
Pulse ≥125	10
Lab findings	
Arterial pH <7.35	30
BUN ≥30 mg/dL	20
Sodium <130 mmol/L	20
Glucose ≥250 mg/dL	10
Ht < 30%	10
PaO2 < 60 mmHg (Pox < 90%)	10
Radiographic finding	
Pleural effusion	10

Risk category (points) and 30-day mortality (%)		
Risk class	Points	30-day mortality (%)
I	0–50	0.1
II	51–70	0.6
III	71–90	0.9
IV	91–130	9.3
V	>130	27.0

Fine et al. [2]; Sligl and Marrie [3]

Table 32.2 CURB-65

	Variable	Point
C	Confusion	1
U	BUN > 7 mmol/L	1
R	RR ≥ 30	1
B	SBP < 90 mmHg or DBP ≤ 60	1
65	Age ≥ 65	1
Risk group (score) and 30-day mortality		
Risk category	Points	30-day mortality (%)
Low	0–1	1.5
Intermediate	2	9.2
High	≥3	22

Lim et al. [4]; Sligl and Marrie [3]

- CURB-65 ≥2 should be admitted to the hospital

SOAR for the elderly? [5]

Severe CAP: 2 criteria: SMART-COP and IDSA/ATS 2007 guide

Table 32.3 SMART-COP

	Variable	Point
S	SBP <90 mmHg	2
M	Multilobar CXR involvement	1
A	Albumin <3.5 d/dL	1
R	RR	1
	Age ≤ 50, RR ≥ 25	
	Age > 50, RR ≥ 30	
T	Tachycardia ≥ 125	1
C	Confusion	1
O	Oxygen	2
	Age ≤ 50, PaO2 < 70 mmHg, Pox ≤ 93% or RI < 333	
	Age > 50, PaO2 < 60 mmHg, Pox ≤ 90%, or RI < 250	
P	Arterial pH < 7.35	2
SMART-COP score and need for MICU care		
Score		Event rate (%)
0		0
1		1.7
2		2.6
3		7.6
4		21.4
5		30.9
6		48.5
≥7		70.8

(continued)

Table 32.3 (continued)

Risk category	
Risk category	Points
Low	0–2
Moderate	3–4
High	5–6
Very high	≥7

- For patients how cannot get albumin, arterial pH or PaO2, skip those items and use following risk stratification

Risk category	Point
Very low	0
Low	1
Moderate	2
High	3
Very high	≥4

Charles et al. [6]

Table 32.4 ICU admission based on IDSA/ATS 2007 guide

• One major or three minor criteria
Major criteria (either one)
Septic shock with need for pressors
Requiring mechanical ventilation
Minor criteria (≥3)
RR ≥ 30
RI ≤ 250
Multilobar infiltrates
Confusion
BUN ≥ 20
WBC < 4000
Platelet < 100,000
Hypothermia <36
Hypotension requiring aggressive fluid resuscitation

Mandel et al. [7]

Approach: Abx, steroid, antiviral?

Table 32.5 Empirical inpatient tx for CAP

β-lactam + macrolide or β-lactam + fluoroquinolone as a base
Add MRSA coverage based on hx and add P. aeruginosa coverage based on hx

Metlay et al. [8]

Aspiration

- CAP patients admitted who had aspiration risks had higher 1-year mortality compared with no risk (HR 1.73) [9]

Table 32.6 Treatment strategy

	CXR +	Clear CXR
Community-acquired	Ampicillin/sulbactam Amoxicillin/clavulanate Fluoroquinolone Carbapenem	Consider bronchoscopy + BAL

Hospital-acquired	MDR risk
	  Risk −: as above
	  Risk +: MDR coverage Zosyn, cefepime + aminoglycoside or colistin
		Consider bronchoscopy + BAL

Mandel and Niederman [10]

- ACEI for prevention? Due to substance P production and promote coughing [10]

Pleural Effusion

- 20–40% of hospitalized pneumonia patients have parapneumonic effusion [11]
- Mortality is much higher in patients with effusion compared with without (RAPID score below)
- Fluid pH $\leq$ 7.20, loculated fluid, large (>50% hemothorax) needs drainage [11]

Effusion Approach [12]

- PNE: RAPID score [13]
- Malignant: LENT score [14]

Three essential information for parapneumonic effusion

1. Septation or loculation
2. Pleural fluid pH $\leq$ 7.20 or not
3. RAPID score $\geq$ 5 or not

Table 32.7 RAPID score

• 3-months mortality	
Variable	Point
Renal (BUN)	
<5	0
5–8	1
>8	2
Age	
<50	0
50–70	1
>70	2
Purulence of pleural fluid	
Purulent	0
Nonpurulent	1
Infection course	
Community acquired	0
Hospital acquired	1
Dietary factor (Albumin g/L)	
≥27	0
<27	1

Risk category	Score	Median survival (days)
Low	0–2	1.4
Moderate	3–4	10.8
High	≥5	43.8

Rahman et al. [13]

Table 32.8 Parapneumonic effusion MGMT

		Septation or loculation	
		No	Yes
pH > 7.2	RAPID < 5	Thoracentesis	Thoracentesis vs chest tube + tPA
	RAPID ≥ 5	Repeat tap vs chest tube	Chest tube + tPA vs VATS
pH ≤7.2	RAPID < 5	Chest tube + tPA	Chest tube + tPA vs VATS
	RAPID ≥ 5	VATS vs chest tube + tPA	VATS vs chest tube + tPA

Feller-Kopman and Right [12]; Anderson et al. [15]

Table 32.9 LENT score

	Variable	Point
L	LDH (IU/L)	
	<1500	0
	>1500	1
E	ECOG PS	
	0	0
	1	1
	2	2
	3–4	3
N	NLR	
	<9	0
	>9	1
T	Tumor type	
	Low risk	0
	Moderate risk	1
	High risk	2

Clive et al. [14]

ECOG PS Eastern Cooperative Oncology Group Performance Score

0   Fully active, able to carry on all pre-disease performance without restriction
1   Restricted in strenuous activity but can carry out light or sedentary work
2   Ambulatory and capable of all selfcare, up and about >50% of waking hours
3   Capable of only limited selfcare, confined to bed or chair >50% of waking hours
4   Completely disabled, cannot carry out any selfcare

NLR neutrophil-to-lymphocyte ratio
Tumor type

Low risk	Mesothelioma
	Hematological malignancy
Moderate	Breast cancer
	Gynecological cancer
	Renal cell carcinoma
High risk	Lung cancer
	Other types

Risk stratification and median survival

Risk category	Score	Median survival (days)
Low	0–1	319
Moderate	2–4	130
High	5–7	44

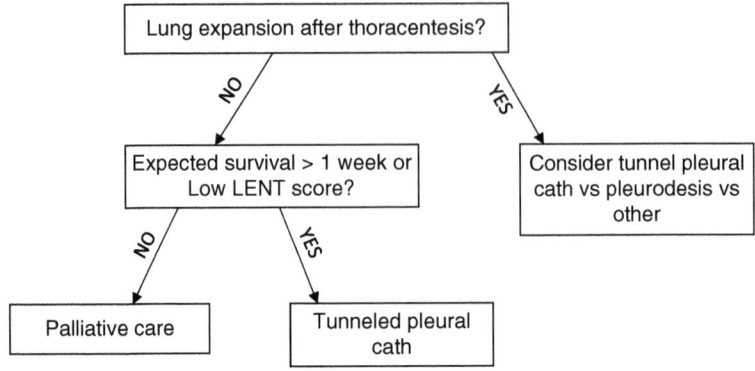

Fig. 32.2 MGMT of malignant effusion [12]

Table 32.10 CVD complication of CAP "Mayo Rule"

Variable	Points
• Cardiac complication occurred in 27% of inpatient [16]	
Variables and points	
Variable	Points
Demographics	
Age	Age in years
PMHx	
CHF	55
CAD	18
Cardiac arrhythmia	18
PE findings	
Pulse	
<80/min	4
>120/min	25
SBP ≥ 140 mmHg or DBP ≥ 90 mmHg	11
Laboratory findings	
Ht < 30%	21
WBC < 12,000/mL	10
Platelet	
<150,000/mL	12
>400,000/mL	17
BUN	
20–40 mg/dL	13
>40 mg/dL	26
Serum glucose >160 mg/dL	18
Arterial pH < 7.35	43
CXR	
Bilateral infiltrates	21
Risk class	
Risk class	Points
I	≤77
II	78–134
III	135–170
IV	171≤

30-day risk of cardiac complication (%)	
Risk class	Cardiac complication (%)
I	5.0
II	8.2
III	28.3
IV	48.9

Corrales-Medina et al. [17]

Table 32.11 Things to consider for non-responders

- It may take 72 h to respond to Abx
- If doesn't respond, then consider the following
  PE
  CHF
  Atypical infection (fungal, parasitic, cryptogenic organizing pneumonia)
  Diffuse alveolar hemorrhage (Vasculitis, pulmonary-renal syndrome)

Povoa et al. [18]

References

1. ☺☺Aliberti S, et al. Community-acquired pneumonia. Lancet. 2021;398:906–19.
2. Fine M, et al. A prediction rule to identify low-risk patients with community-acquired pneumonia. N Engl J Med. 1997;336:243–50.
3. Sligl W, Marrie T. Severe community-acquired pneumonia. Crit Care Clin. 2013;29:563–601.
4. Lim W, et al. Defining community acquired pneumonia severity on presentation to hospital: an international derivation and validation study. Thorax. 2003;58:377–82.
5. Myint P, et al. Severity assessment criteria recommended by the British Thoracic Society (VTS) for community-acquired pneumonia (CAP) and older patients. Should SOAR (systolic blood pressure, oxygenation, age and respiratory rate) criteria be used in older people? A compilation study of two prospective cohorts. Age Ageing. 2006;35:286–91.
6. ☺Charles P, et al. SMART-COP: a tool for predicting the need for intensive respiratory or vasopressor support in community-acquired pneumonia. Clin Infect Dis. 2008;47:375–87.
7. Mandell L, et al. Infectious Disease Society of America/American Thoracic Society consensus guidelines on the management of community-acquired pneumonia in adults. Clin Infect Dis. 2007;44:S27–72.
8. ☺☺Metlay J, et al. Diagnosis and treatment of adults with community-acquired pneumonia. Am J Respir Crit Care Med. 2019;200(7):e45–67.
9. Taylor J, et al. Risk factors for aspiration in community-acquired pneumonia: analysis of a hospitalized UK cohort. Am J Med. 2013;126:995–1001.
10. ☺Mandell L, Niederman M. Aspiration pneumonia. N Engl J Med. 2019;380:651–63.
11. ☺☺Light R. Parapneumonic effusions and empyema. Proc Am Thorac Soc. 2006;3:75–80.
12. ☺☺Feller-Kopman D, Light R. Pleural disease. N Engl J Med. 2018;378:740–51.
13. Rahman N, et al. A clinical score (RAPID) to identify those at risk for poor outcome at presentation in patients with pleural infection. Chest. 2014;145(4):848–55.
14. Clive A, et al. Predicting survival in malignant pleural effusion: development and validation of the LENT prognostic score. Thorax. 2014;69:1098–104.

15. ☺ ☺ Anderson D, et al. Comprehensive review of chest tube management. A review. JAMA Surg. 2022;157(3):269–74.
16. Corrales-Medina V, et al. Acute pneumonia and the cardiovascular system. Lancet. 2013;381:496–505.
17. ☺ ☺ ☺ Corrales-Medina V, et al. Risk stratification for cardiac complications in patients hospitalized for community-acquired pneumonia. Mayo Clin Proc. 2014;89(1):60–8.
18. ☺ Povoa P, et al. How to approach a patient hospitalized for pneumonia who is not responding to treatment? Intensive Care Med. 2025;51:893–903.

Asthma/COPD

33

Asthma

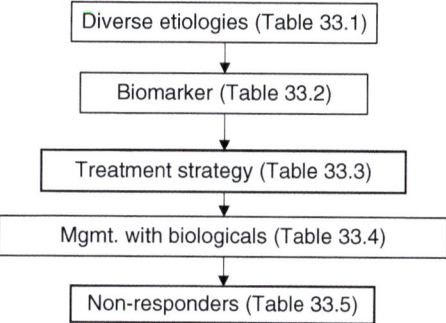

Table 33.1 Diverse etiology

T2 high		T2 low
Allergic asthma (ICS sensitive)	Eosinophilic asthma	(ICS resistant)
Alarmins (IL-33, IL-25, TSLP (thymic stromal lymphopoietin))		
Th2	ILC2 (GATA3)	Th1, Th17
IL-4, IL-5, IL-13	IL-5, IL-13, CRTH2	IL-6, IL-17 TNF, interferon
Mast cell	Eosinophils	Neutrophil
B cell		
Eosinophils		
Eosinophil counts in blood/sputum		
FeNO		
Periostin concentration [1]		

Modified from Bel and ten Brinke [2]; Israel and Reddel [3]; Brusselle and Koppelman [4]

Table 33.2 Biomarker

Biomarker	Cutoff
IgE	Variable
Blood eosinophil count	$\geq 0.15 \times 10^9/L$
Sputum eosinophil	$\geq 2\%$
FENO	≥ 25 ppb

Couillard et al. [5]

- NO is a product of T2 airway inflammation and produced by airway epithelial cells as a result of IL-13 induced induction of NO synthase.
- Blood eosinophil + FeNo are the most practical and helpful biomarkers to determine lower airway inflammatory phenotype and ICS responsiveness

Mgmt

- ICS is the cornerstone of asthma mgmt [6]

Table 33.3 Expert panel report (EPR)-3

Step	Meds
• LAMA can be used for long term but NOT in ED or inpatient settings	
1	SABA PRN
2	Low ICS + SABA PRN
3	Low ICS + LABA QD + PRN
	Low ICS + LAMA QD + SABA PRN
4	Medium ICS + LABA QD
	Medium ICS + LAMA QD + SABA PRN
5	Medium-high ICS + LABA + LAMA QD + SABA PRN
6	High ICS + LABA + oral steroid + SABA PRN

Reddel et al. [7]; Cloutier et al. [8]

Severe asthma and difficult to treat asthma strategy

Table 33.4 Biological therapy for asthma

• Difficult to treat asthma obtain blood eosinophil count and FENO	
• TSLP: thymic stromal lymphopoietin is one of airway alarmins	
FENO < 25	FENO ≥ 25
Eos < 150/µL	Eos ≥ 150–300/µL
T2-Lo disease	T2-Hi disease
Anti-TSLP	Anti-IgE
	Anti-IL-4
	Anti IL-5, 5R

Peters and Wenzel [1]; Brusselle and Koppelman [9];Wenzel [10]

Table 33.5 Things to consider for non-responders

1. PE
2. CHF
3. Atypical infection
4. Vocal cord dysfunction

COPD

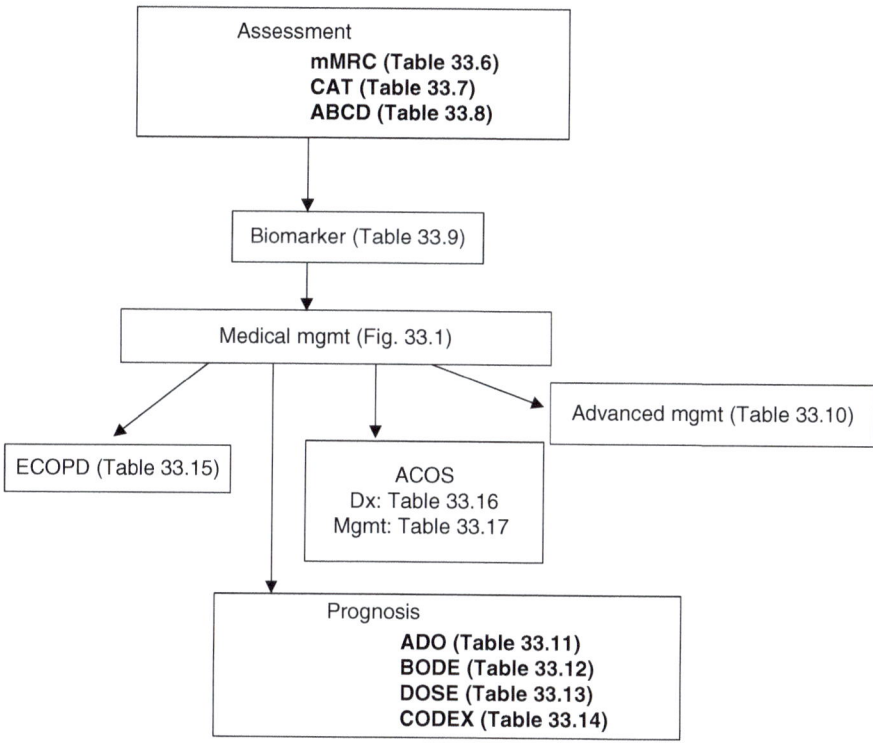

FACTS:

- COPD is a systemic chronic inflammatory disease [11–13]
- COPD treatment approach by endotyping/biomarkers [13]
- Endotype biomarkers: alpha tripsin (AAT), neutrophil elastase (NE) [14] and blood eosinophil counts [15]

SCALES:

- Airway obstruction: GOLD stage def: FEV1/FVC < 0.7
- But airway obstruction doesn't predict severity and disability mMRC, CAT

Table 33.6 mMRC dyspnea scale

Grade	Definition
1	Not troubled by breathlessness except on strenuous exercise
2	SOB when hurrying or walking up a slight hill
3	Walks slower than cotemporaries on level ground due to SOB or has to stop for breath when walking at own pace
4	Stops for breath after walking about 100 m or after a few minutes on level ground
5	Too breathless to leave the house, or breathless when dressing or undressing

Conway et al. [16]

Table 33.7 CAT (COPD assessment test)

• 5 is the worst degree in each variable	
• Health status evaluation for COPD patients	
Variable	Point
Cough	1–5
Amount of phlegm	1–5
Chest tightness	1–5
Walk up one flight of stairs or hill breathless	1–5
Limited doing any activities at home	1–5
Confident leaving home despite lung condition	1–5
Sleep soundly	1–5
Energy	1–5

Jones et al. [17]

Table 33.8 ABCD assessment tool

GOLD stage	FEV1
1	≥80
2	50–79
3	30–49
4	<30

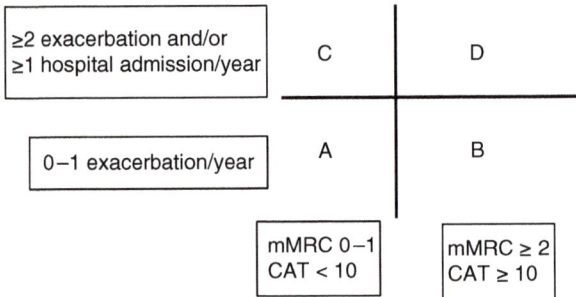

Vogelmeier et al. [18]

Table 33.9 Biomarkers

- Phenotype marker: CT chest, DLco
- Endotype marker: Alpha1 antitrypsin and blood eosinophil count (BEC)
- Neutrophil elastase (NE)

Celli and Wedzicha [15]; Stockley [14]

Fig. 33.1 Medical mgmt [19]

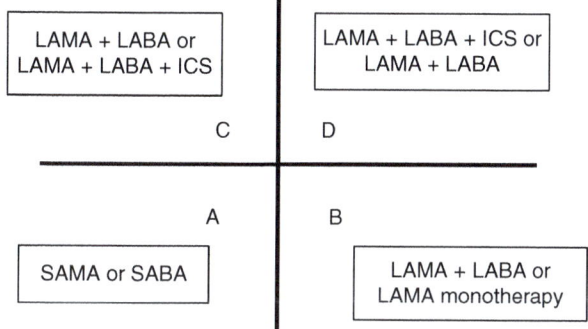

Further Treatment

- Blood eosinophil count (BEC) predicts the response to ICS.
- GOLD 2019 recommended blood eosinophil counts as part of a precision medicine strategy.
- Higher BEC are associated with higher concentrations of T2 inflammation markers in the airways [15, 20]

  >300 good response
  100–300 moderate response
  <100 minimal benefit

- Macrolides Abx
- Phosphodiesterase-4 inhibitor (PDE4i) roflumilast
- Supplementary O2
- If no exacerbation in 1 year, take out ICS from triple to maintain LAMA + LABA [21]

Table 33.10 Advanced mgmt

Emphysema with severe hyperinflation		No candidate for bullectomy, BLVR or LVRS
Bulla ++	No bulla	
Bullectomy	Bronchoscopic lung volume reduction (BLVR) Lung volume reduction surgery (LVRS)	Lung transplant

Vogelmeier et al. [18]

Prognosis

Table 33.11 ADO score

Variable	Point
• Predicts 3-year mortality	
• Based on age, dyspnea and airway obstruction	
FEV1 (% predicted)	
≥81	0
65–80	1
51–64	2
36–50	3
≤35	4
Dyspnea (mMRC)	
0	0
1–2	1
3	2
4	3
Age	
40–49	0
50–59	2
60–69	4
70–79	5
≥80	7

3-year mortality (%) based on updated ADO score														
	0	1	2	3	4	5	6	7	8	9	10	11	12	13	14
Mortality (%)	0.7	1.0	1.6	2.3	3.4	4.9	7.2	10.3	14.5	20.1	27.2	35.7	45.1	55.0	64.5

Puhan et al. [22]; Puhan (2012)

Table 33.12 BODE score

	Variable	Point
• Survival up to 52 months		
B	BMI	
	>21	0
	≤21	1
O	Obstruction FEV1 (%predicted)	
	≥65	0
	50–64	1
	36–49	2
	≤35	3
D	Dyspnea (mMRC scale)	
	0–1	0
	2	1
	3	2
	4	3
E	Exercise capacity (6-min walk (m))	
	≥350	0
	250–349	1
	150–249	2
	≤149	3

• Risk quartile (score) and 52 months mortality		
Risk category quartile	BODE score	Mortality (%)
1	0–2	20
2	3–4	30
3	5–6	45
4	7–10	80

Celli and Cote [23]

Table 33.13 DOSE score

• Predict risk of hospital admission		
• Score ≥ 4 had greater risk of hospital admission and respiratory failure		
	Variable	Point
D	Dyspnea (mMRC scale)	
	0–1	0
	2	1
	3	2
	4	3
O	Obstruction (FEV1% predicted)	
	>50	0
	30–49	1
	<30	2
S	Smoking status	
	Nonsmoker	0
	Smoker	1
E	Exacerbation frequency per year	
	0–1	0
	2–3	1
	>3	2

Jones et al. [24]

Table 33.14 CODEX score

	Variable	Point
C	Comorbidity (Charlson index)	
	0–4	0
	5–7	1
	≥8	2
O	Obstruction FEV1%	
	≥65	0
	50–64	1
	36–49	2
	≤35	3
D	Dyspnea (mMRC scale)	
	0–1	0
	2	1
	3	2
	4	3
EX	Exacerbation	
	0	0
	1–2	1
	≥3	2

Risk category and 1 year mortality		
Risk category	Score	Mortality (%)
Low	0–4	<10
High	≥5	20

Almagro et al. [25]

ECOPD

COPD exacerbation (ECOPD) [26]

- CRP > 10 mg/L as a marker
- DDx for ECOPD
    1. HF
    2. PE
    3. Pneumonia

Four exacerbation clusters [27]
1. High TNF and IL-1β
2. High CXCL10 and CXCL 11
3. High CCL17 and IL-5
4. Pauci-inflammatory biomarkers

Table 33.15 Severity of ECOPD

Mild	Moderate (at least 3 out of 5)	Severe
Dyspnea (visual analog scale <5) RR < 24 HR < 95 Pox(RA) ≥ 92% CRP < 10 mg/L	Dyspnea VAS ≥ 5 RR ≥ 24 HR ≥ 95 Pox (RA) < 92% CRP ≥ 10	ABG PaCO2 > 45 mmHg and pH < 7.35

Table 33.16 Asthma-COPD overlap (ACO)

Criteria: all 4 major + at least 1 minor are present	
Major	Minor
1. Age ≥ 40 2. Post bronchodilator FEV1/FVC < 0.7 3. Exposure ≥10 pack-years of tobacco or equivalent air pollution 4. Asthma <40 y/o or bronchodilator response of >400 mL in FEV1	1. Allergic rhinitis or atopic disease 2. Bronchodilator response ≥200 mL and 12% from baseline values on ≥2 encounters 3. Blood eosinophil counts ≥300/µL

Maselli et al. [28]

Table 33.17 Tx strategy

	COPD	ACO	Asthma
Initial therapy	LABA or LAMA	ICS	ICS
Escalation	LAMA + LABA	ICS + LABA	ICS + LABA
Advanced therapy	LAMA + LABA + ICS		
Escalation	Roflumilast (PDE4i) macrolides	Monoclonal Abx (anti-IgE, anti-IL5)	

References

1. Peters M, Wenzel S. Intersection of biology and therapeutics: type 2 targeted therapeutics for adult asthma. Lancet. 2020;395:371–83.
2. Bel E, ten Brinke A. New anti-eosinophil drugs for asthma and COPD. Targeting the trait! Chest. 2017;152(6):1276–82.
3. ☺☺Israel E, Reddel H. Severe and difficult-to-treat asthma in adults. N Engl J Med. 2017;377:965–76.
4. ☺☺☺Brusselle G, Koppelman G. Biologic therapies for severe asthma. N Engl J Med. 2022;386:157–71.
5. Couillard S, et al. Workup of severe asthma. Chest. 2021;160(6):2019–29.
6. ☺Yawn B, Han M. Practical considerations for the diagnosis and management of asthma in older adults. Mayo Clin Proc. 2017;92(11):1697–705.
7. Reddel H, et al. Global initiative for asthma strategy 2021. Executive summary and rationale for key changes. Am J Respir Crit Care Med. 2022;205(1):17–35.

8. ☺☺Cloutier M, et al. Managing asthma in adolescents and adults. 2020 asthma guideline update from the national asthma education and prevention program. JAMA. 2020;324(22):2301–17.

9. Brusselle G, Koppelman G. Biologic therapies for severe asthma. N Engl J Med. 2022;386:157–71.

10. Wenzel S. Severe adult asthmas: integrating clinical features, biology, and therapeutics to improve outcomes. Am J Respir Crit Care Med. 2021;203(7):809–21.

11. Fabbri L, Rabe K. From COPD to chronic systemic inflammatory syndrome? Lancet. 2007;370:797–9.

12. ☺☺☺Polverino F, et al. COPD: to be or not to be, that is the question. Am J Med. 2019;132:1271–8.

13. ☺☺☺Agusti A, et al. Chronic obstructive pulmonary disease 1. What does endotyping mean for treatment in chronic obstructive pulmonary disease? Lancet. 2017;390:980–7.

14. Stockley R, et al. Chronic obstructive pulmonary disease biomarkers and their interpretation. Am J Respir Crit Care Med. 2019;199(10):1195–204.

15. ☺☺Celli B, Wedzicha J. Update on clinical aspects of chronic obstructive pulmonary disease. N Engl J Med. 2019;381:1257–66.

16. Conway F, et al. Diagnosing chronic obstructive pulmonary disease. BMJ. 2015;351:h6171. https://doi.org/10.1136/bmj.h6171.

17. Jones P, et al. Development and first validation of the COPD assessment test. Eur Respir J. 2009;34:648–54.

18. Vogelmeier C, et al. Global strategy for the diagnosis, management, and prevention of chronic obstructive lung disease 2017 report. GOLD executive summary. Am J Respir Crit Care Med. 2017;195(5):557–82.

19. Riley C, Sciurba F. Diagnosis and outpatient management of chronic obstructive pulmonary disease. A review. JAMA. 2019;321(8):786–97.

20. ☺Singh D, et al. Blood eosinophils and chronic obstructive pulmonary disease. A global initiative for chronic obstructive lung disease science committee 2022 review. Am J Respir Crit Care Med. 2022;206(1):17–24.

21. Nici L, et al. Pharmacologic management of chronic obstructive pulmonary disease. An official American Thoracic Society clinical practice guideline. Am J Respir Crit Care Med. 2020;201(9):e56–69.

22. Puhan M, et al. Expansion of the prognostic assessment of patients with chronic obstructive pulmonary disease: the updated BODE index and the ADO index. Lancet. 2009;374:704–11.

23. Celli B, Cote C. The body-mass index, airflow obstruction, dyspnea, and exercise capacity index in chronic obstructive pulmonary disease. N Engl J Med. 2004;350:1005–12.

24. Jones R, et al. Derivation and validation of a composite index of severity in chronic obstructive pulmonary disease. The DOSE index. Am J Respir Crit Care Med. 2009;180:1189–95.

25. ☺Almagro P, et al. Short- and medium-term prognosis in patients hospitalized for COPD exacerbation. The CODEX index. Chest. 2014;145(5):972–80.

26. Celli B, et al. An updated definition and severity classification of chronic obstructive pulmonary disease exacerbations. The Rome proposal. Am J Respir Crit Care Med. 2021;204(11):1251–8.

27. ☺☺☺Christenson S, et al. Chronic obstructive pulmonary disease. Lancet. 2022;399:2227–42.

28. ☺Maselli D, et al. Clinical approach to the therapy of asthma-COPD overlap. Chest. 2019;155(1):168–77.

Acute Pancreatitis

34

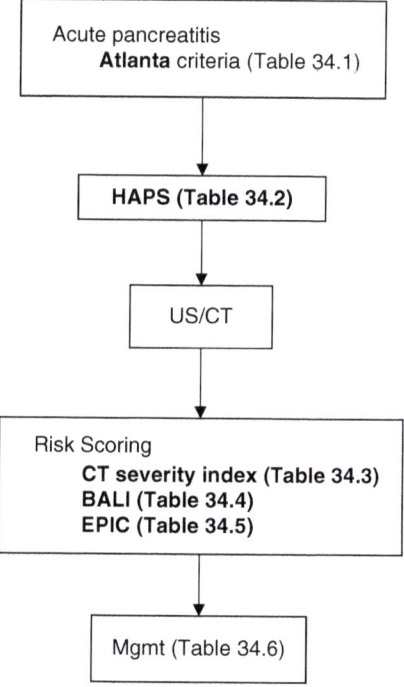

Diagnosis:

Table 34.1 Atlanta criteria

1. Abdominal pain consistent with acute pancreatitis
2. Elevated serum amylase or lipase > ×3 ULN
3. Characteristic findings of acute pancreatitis on imaging

Banks et al. [1]

Table 34.2 HAPS (the harmless acute pancreatitis score)

Presence of the following three parameters predict non-severe course:

No rebound tenderness/guarding,

Serum creatinine ≤ 2 mg/dL,

Ht normal.

Lankisch et al. [2]

Scoring:

Table 34.3 CT severity index

CT severity index = CT grade points + %Necrosis points	
Variable	Points
CT grade	
A: normal	0
B: enlarged	1
C: peripancreatic inflammation and/or peripancreatic fat	2
D: a single peripancreatic fluid collection	3
E: at least two fluid collection and/or retroperitoneal air	4
%Necrosis	
0	0
<30	2
30–50	4
>50	6

Severity index and outcome		
Severity index	Mortality (%)	Morbidity (%)
0–1	0	0
2	0	4
7–10	17	92

Balthazar [3]

Table 34.4 BALI

Variables: BALI	
BUN ≥ 25 mg/dL	
Age ≥ 65	
LDH ≥ 300 IU/L	
IL-6 ≥ 300 pg/mL	
Risk score and outcome	
Risk score	Mortality (%)
0	0
≤2	5
3	27
4	54

Spitzer et al. [4]

Table 34.5 EPIC score

• Examining four extra-pancreatic signs of inflammation	
Variable	Point
Pleural effusion	
None	0
Unilateral	1
Bilateral	2
Ascites in either of four locations: perisplenic, perihepatic, interloop or pelvis	
None	0
One location	1
>1 locations	2
Retroperitoneal inflammation	
None	0
Unilateral	1
Bilateral	2
Mesenteric inflammation	
None	0
Present	1
Score	Mortality (%)
0–3	0
7	67

De Waele et al. [5]

Table 34.6 MGMT

Fluid: LR 3 mL/kg/h as a guide to maintain HR < 120, UO > 1 mL/kg/h, Ht 35–44%
Nutrition: as soon as tolerated, NG tube if oral intolerance in 3–5 days
GB stone pancreatitis: cholecystectomy in first admission

Mederos et al. [6]

References

1. Banks P, et al. Classification of acute pancreatitis – 2012: revision of the Atlanta classification and definitions by international consensus. Gut. 2013;62:102–11.
2. Lankisch P, et al. The harmless acute pancreatitis score: a clinical algorithm for rapid initial stratification of nonsevere disease. Clin Gastroenterol Hepatol. 2009;7:702–5.
3. Balthazar E. Acute pancreatitis: assessment of severity with clinical and CT evaluation. Radiology. 2002;223:603–13.
4. Spitzer A, et al. Applying Ockham's razor to pancreatitis prognostication. A four-variable predictive model. Ann Surg. 2006;243:380–8.
5. De Waele J, et al. Extrapancreatic inflammation on abdominal computed tomography as an early predictor of disease severity in acute pancreatitis. Evaluation of a new scoring system. Pancreas. 2007;34:185–90.
6. ☺ ☺ ☺ Mederos M, et al. Acute pancreatitis. A review. JAMA. 2021;325(4):382–90.

GI Bleeding

35

General

- According to the ACG bleeding registry, 76% of GI bleeding are from upper GI bleed (UGIB) and 45.5% of GI bleeding received endoscopy [1]
- About 11% of lower GI bleed (LGIB) are secondary to UGIB [2]
- LGIB is slower and less massive than UGIB due to arterial anatomy. Spontaneous cessative of bleeding occur >80% of cases [2]
- Validated risk scores are only available for UPPER GI bleeding [3]

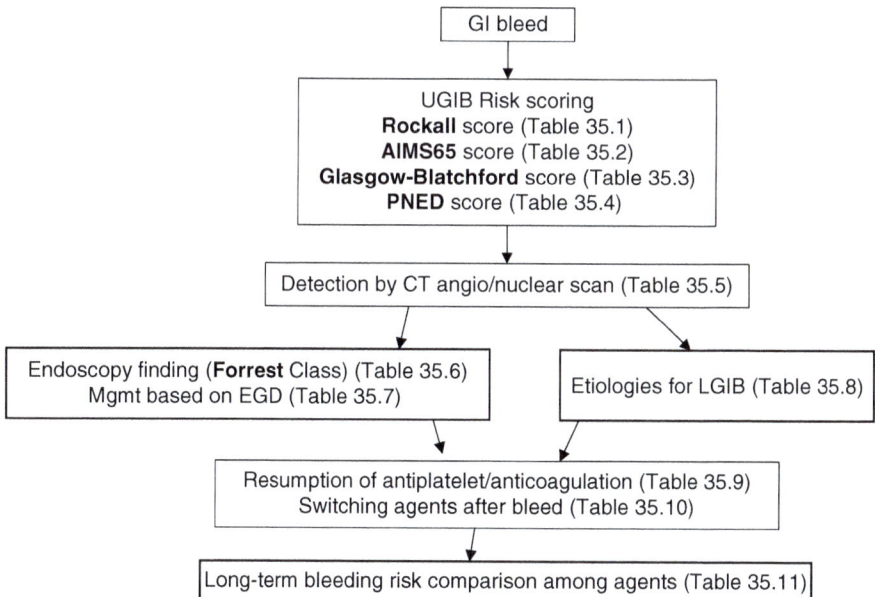

© The Author(s), under exclusive license to Springer Nature Switzerland AG 2025
M. J. Morikawa, *The Inpatient Medicine Handbook*,
https://doi.org/10.1007/978-3-032-08398-2_35

Risk Scores

Rockall score = rebleed and mortality

AIMS65 score = in-hospital mortality

Glasgow-Blatchford score = outpatient mgmt or not

PNED score = 30-day mortality

Table 35.1 Rockall score

variable	Point
Age	
<60	0
60–79	1
≥80	2
Shock	
SBP ≥ 100, pulse < 100	0
SBP ≥ 100, pulse ≥ 100	1
SBP < 100	2
Comorbidity	
No major comorbidity	0
Cardiac failure, ischemic heart disease, any major comorbidity	2
Renal failure, liver failure, disseminated malignancy	3
Diagnosis	
Mallory-Weiss tear, no lesion identified and no SRH	0
All other diagnosis	1
Malignancy of upper GI tract	2
Major stigmata of recent hemorrhage	
None or dark spot only	0
Blood in upper GI tract, adherent clot visible or spurting vessel	2

Score and outcome (%)									
	0	1	2	3	4	5	6	7	≥8
Rebleed (%)	4.9	3.4	5.3	11.2	14.1	24.1	32.9	43.8	41.8
Mortality (%)	0	0	0.2	2.9	5.3	10.8	17.3	27.0	41.1

Rockall et al. [4]; Wilkins et al. [5]

Table 35.2 AIMS65

• Predict in-hospital mortality due to Upper GI bleeding		
	Variable	Point
A	Albumin < 3.0 g/dL	1
I	INR > 1.5	1
M	Altered mental status	1
S	SBP ≤ 90 mmHg	1
65	Age > 65	1

Score and in-hospital mortality (%)					
	0	1	2	3	4	5
Mortality (%)	0.3	1.2	2.8	8.5	15.1	24.5

Saltzman et al. [6]

Table 35.3 Glasgow-Blatchford score (GBS)

• Identify low risk upper GI bleeding patient suitable for outpatient mgmt	
Variable	Point
BUN (mmol/L)	
6.5–7.9	2
8.0–9.9	3
10.0–25.0	4
≥25.0	6
Hb for men (g/dL)	
12–12.9	1
10–11.9	3
<10.0	6
Hb for women (g/dL)	
10.0–11.9	1
<10.0	6
SBP (mmHg)	
100–109	1
90–99	2
<90	3
Other markers	
Pulse ≥100	1
Presentation with melena	1
Presentation with syncope	2
Liver disease Hx	2
CHF Hx	2
• GBS = 0: outpatient mgmt.	
GBS = 0	
Urea < 6.5 mmol/L	
Hb ≥ 13 mg/dL (men), ≥12 mg/dL (women)	
SBP ≥ 110 mmHg	
Pulse < 100	
Absence of melena, syncope, liver disease or CHF	

Stanley et al. [7]

Table 35.4 PNED score

• UGIB for 30-day mortality	
Point	Risk factors
1	ASA3
	Time to admission < 8 h
2	Hb ≤ 7 g/dL
	Age ≥ 80
	Renal failure
3	Rebleeding
	ASA4
	Neoplasm
	Liver cirrhosis
4	Failure of endoscopic treatment

ASA3	ASA4
Non life threatening systemic diseases ≥1 of the following:	Severe systemic disease constant threat to life
Poorly controlled HTN or DM	Recent (<3 month) MI or CVA
Obesity (BMI ≥ 40)	Not regularly scheduled HD
CKD, regularly scheduled HD, COPD	

Risk category (points) and 30-day mortality		
Risk category	Score	Mortality (%)
Low	0–4	<5
Medium	5–8	10
High	≥9	32

Marmo et al. [8]

Diagnosis/Etiologies

BUN/Cr ratio?

Endoscopy

Table 35.5 Bleeding detection by CT angio vs radionuclide scintigraphy

CT angiography	Radionuclide scintigraphy
As low as 0.3 mL/min of bleeding	As low as 0.1 mL/min of bleeding

Gralnek et al. [9]

Upper GI

• INR <2.5 before endoscope [7]

Table 35.6 Forrest classification

Active bleeding Forrest I	Recent bleeding Forrest II	No evidence of bleeding Forrest III
Spurting (Ia) Oozing blood (Ib)	Visible protruding artery (IIa) Adherent clot (IIb) Flat pigmented spot (IIc)	Clean ulcer base (III)

Rebleeding risk after endoscopy based on Forrest class					
	Active bleeding (Forrest I)	Visible artery (Forrest IIa)	Adherent clot (Forrest IIb)	Flat pigmented spot (Forrest IIc)	No bleeding (Forrest III)
Rebleeding rate (%)	55	43	22	10	5

Forrest et al. [10]; Lau et al. [11]; Kamboj et al. [12]

Table 35.7 UGIB mgmt based on EGD findings

EGD finding	Active bleeding or visible artery (Forrest I and IIa)	Adherent clot (Forrest IIb)	Flat pigmented spot (Forrest IIc)	Clean base (Forrest III)
EGD tx	Yes	Maybe	No	No
PPI	Intensive PPI	Intensive PPI	Oral PPI QD	Oral PPI QD
Diet	Clear liquid × 2 days	Clear liquid × 2 day	Clear liquid × 1 day	Regular diet
Disposition	Hospitalize × 3 days	3 days	1–2 days	Discharge after EGD

Laine and Jensen [13]; Laine [14]

- Intensive PPI: 80 mg IV with 8 mg/h DIV × 72 h or 80 mg IV + 80 mg PO BID × 3 days

Table 35.8 LGIB etiologies

Etiology	Frequency (%)
Diverticulosis	30–65
Ischemic colitis	5–20
Hemorrhoids	5–20
Colorectal polyps or neoplasms	2–15
Angioectasias	5–10

Gralnek et al. [9]

Table 35.9 When to reintroduce antiplatelet/anticoagulation?

ASA	ASAP or <3 days
DAPT	ASA ASAP, P2Y12 < 5–7 days
VKA	<7 days with higher rebleeding risk
	Resume 7–15 days if high VTE risk, bridge with LMWH day 2–7
DOAC	As soon as hemostasis vs day 3

Chan et al. [15]; Sung et al. [16]; Scott et al. [17]; Gralnek et al. [18]

Table 35.10 Switching agents after bleeding

Agent before bleed	VKA	Dabigatran/ rivaroxaban	Apixaban	DAPT or ASA with anticoagulant
Strategy	VKA/Strict INR Apixaban	VKA/Strict INR Apixaban	VKA/Strict INR Apixaban 2.5 bid	Single antiplatelet

Scott et al. [17]

Table 35.11 Long-term bleeding risk comparison among agents

ASA	Clopidogrel	VKA	ASA + Clopidogrel	ASA + VKA	Clopidogrel + VKA	ASA + Clopidogrel + VKA
1.0	1.33	1.23	1.47	1.84	3.52	4.05

Warfarin	ASA	Clopidogrel	ASA + Clopidogrel	Warfarin + ASA	Clopidogrel + warfarin	ASA + Clopidogrel + VKA
1.0	0.93	1.06	1.66	1.83	3.08	3.70

Sorensen et al. [19]; Hansen et al. [20]

References

1. Peura D, et al. The American College of Gastroenterology bleeding registry: preliminary findings. Am J Gastroenterol. 1997;92(6):924–8.
2. Qayed E, et al. Lower gastrointestinal hemorrhage. Crit Care Clin. 2016;32:241–54.
3. Palmer K, Nairn M. Management of acute gastrointestinal blood loss: summary of SIGN guidelines. BMJ. 2008;337:928–30.
4. Rockall T, et al. Risk assessment after acute upper gastrointestinal haemorrhage. Gut. 1996;38:316–21.
5. Wilkins T, et al. Diagnosis and management of upper gastrointestinal bleeding. Am Fam Physician. 2012;85(5):469–76.
6. ☺☺Saltzman J, et al. A simple risk score accurately predicts in-hospital mortality, length of stay, and cost in acute upper GI bleeding. Gastrointest Endosc. 2011;74:1215–24.
7. Stanley A, et al. Outpatient management of patients with low-risk upper-gastrointestinal haemorrhage: multicentre validation and prospective evaluation. Lancet. 2009;373:42–7.
8. Marmo R, et al. Predicting mortality in non-variceal upper gastrointestinal bleeders: validation of the Italian PNED score and prospective comparison with the Rockall score. Am J Gastroenterol. 2010;105:1284–91.
9. ☺☺☺Gralnek I, et al. Acute lower gastrointestinal bleeding. N Engl J Med. 2017;376:1054–63.
10. ☺Forrest J, et al. Endoscopy in gastrointestinal bleeding. Lancet. 1974;304:394–7.
11. ☺☺Lau J, et al. Challenges in the management of acute peptic ulcer bleeding. Lancet. 2013;381:2033–43.
12. Kamboj A, et al. Upper gastrointestinal bleeding: etiologies and management. Mayo Clin Proc. 2019;94(4):697–703.
13. Laine L, Jensen D. Management of patients with ulcer bleeding. Am J Gastroenterol. 2012;107:345–60.
14. ☺☺☺Laine L. Upper gastrointestinal bleeding due to a peptic ulcer. N Engl J Med. 2016;374:2367–76.

15. Chan F, et al. Management of patients on antithrombotic agents undergoing emergency and elective endoscopy: joint Asian Pacific Association of Gastroenterology (APAGE) and Asian Pacific Society of Digestive Endoscopy (APSDE) practice guidelines. Gut. 2018;67:405–17.
16. Sung J, et al. Asia-Pacific working group consensus on non-variceal upper gastrointestinal bleeding: an update 2018. Gut. 2018;67:1757–68.
17. Scott M, et al. Reintroduction of anti-thrombotic therapy after a gastrointestinal haemorrhage: if and when? Br J Haematol. 2017;177:185–97.
18. Gralnek I, et al. Diagnosis and management of nonvariceal upper gastrointestinal hemorrhage: European Society of Gastrointestinal Endoscopy (ESGE) guideline. Endoscopy. 2015;47:1–46.
19. ☺☺Sorensen R, et al. Risk of bleeding in patients with acute myocardial infraction treated with different combinations of aspirin, clopidogrel, and vitamin K antagonists in Denmark: a retrospective analysis of nationwide registry data. Lancet. 2009;374:1967–74.
20. Hansen M, et al. Risk of bleeding with single, dual, or triple therapy with warfarin, aspirin, and clopidogrel in patients with atrial fibrillation. Arch Intern Med. 2010;170(16):1433–41.

Diarrhea

36

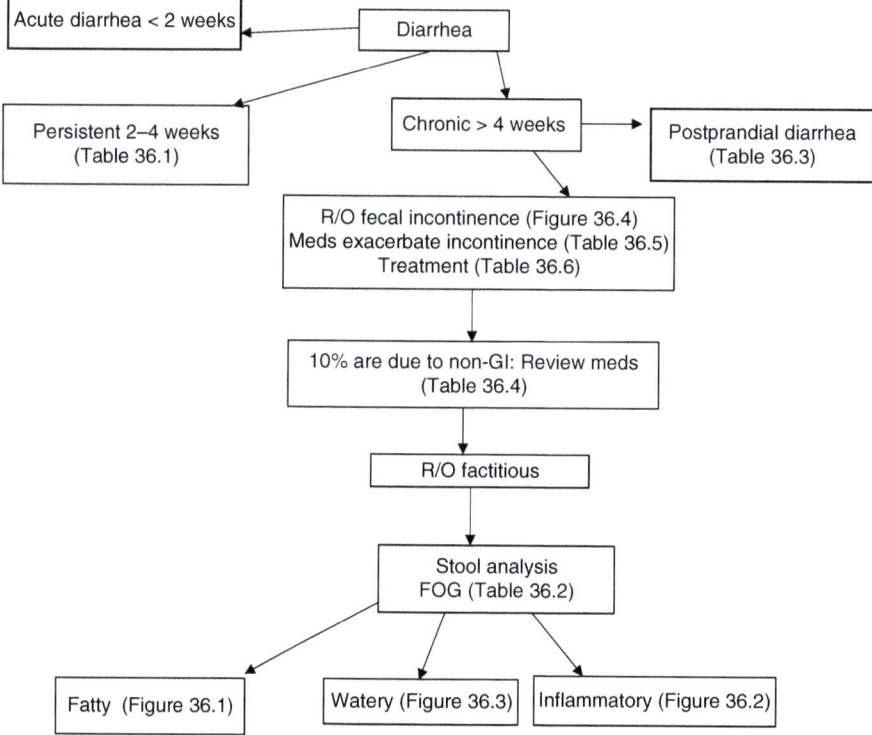

- Acute <2 weeks: mostly infectious and usually subsides <2 weeks [1, 2]
- Persistent diarrhea (>14 days)
- Parasites, protozoae, infection, recurrent infection (CDI) or noninfectious causes (lactase deficiency, postinfectious IBS)

Table 36.1 Persistent diarrhea

Abdominal pain/ discomfort	Recent hospital stay or NH stay	Travel to developing countries	Blood or mucus in stools
Stool cx, parasite screen Evaluate for IBS, IBD, ischemic colitis	Check for CDI	Treat with azithromycin 1000 mg × once Then stool cx, parasites	Stool parasite, stool culture

DuPont [3]

Chronic Diarrhea (>4 weeks)
- Basic pathophysiology of diarrhea is "Incomplete absorption of water from the lumen" [4].
  1. Watery, Osmotic and secretory
  2. Fatty
  3. Inflammatory
- Watery diarrhea:
  1. Secretory—reduced rate of net water absorption FOG low neuroendocrine tumor can be a cause of secretory diarrhea [5].
  2. Osmotic—Osmotic retention of water intraluminally due to the presence of poorly absorbed substances FOG high [6–9].

Table 36.2 FOG: fecal osmotic gap

FOG = 290 – 2 (Na + K)
High: FOG > 50 mOsm/kg—Osmotic diarrhea
Low: FOG < 50 mOsm/kg—Secretory diarrhea

Carollo and Schiller [4]

Fatty diarrhea:

- Steatorrhea, identified by Sudan stain, quantitative fat analysis.

Inflammatory diarrhea:
- Associated with blood and pus
- Fecal leukocyte count is elevated
- In reality, classification of osmotic vs secretory is not distinctive, since some of the pathologies may have both components depending on the severity of disease.
- The distinction and classification will incorporate enteric hormones and based on intestinal endocrine cells [10].

Table 36.3 Postprandial diarrhea

- Pancreatic exocrine insufficiency
- Glucosidase inhibition and deficiency
- Bile acid malabsorption

Money and Camilleri [11]

Table 36.4 Medications causing diarrhea

• ACEI [7]	
Mechanism	Drugs
Osmotic	Citrate, phosphates, sulfates
	Magnesium-containing antacids/laxatives
	Sugar alcohols
Secretory	Antiarrhythmics (quinine)
	Antibiotics
	Biguanides
	Digitalis
	Colchicine
	NSAID
	Prostaglandins
Motility	Macrolides
	Metoclopramide
	Stimulant laxatives
Malabsorption	Acarbose
	Aminoglycosides
	Ticlopidine
Pseudomembranous colitis	Antibiotics
	Immunosuppressants

Burgers et al. [6]; Jucket and Trivedi [8]

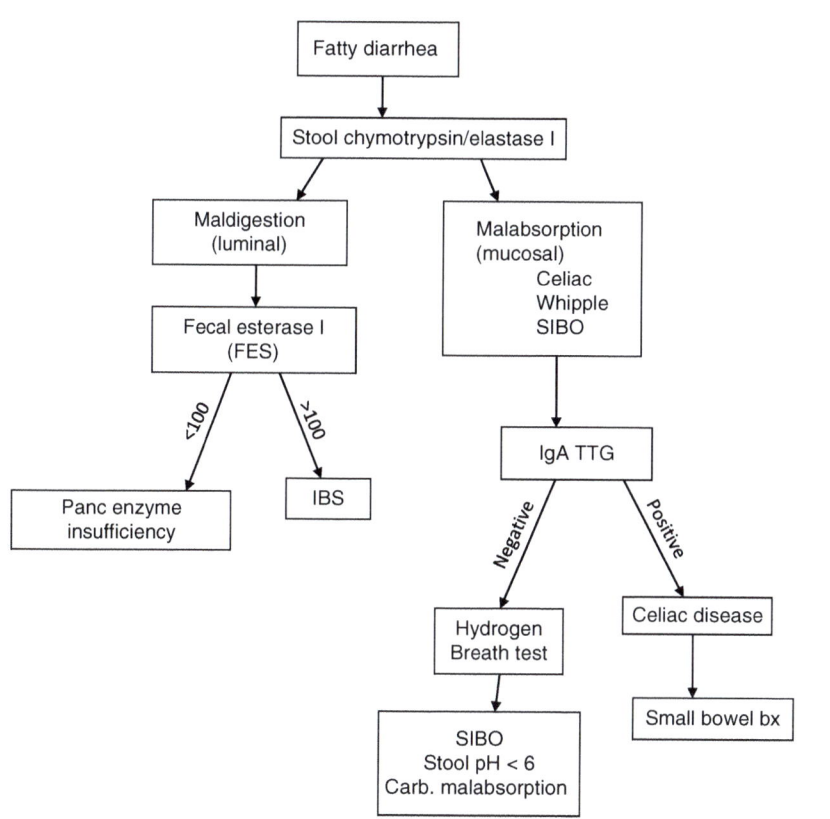

Fig. 36.1 Fatty diarrhea

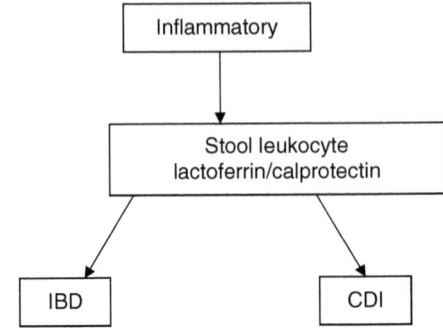

Fig. 36.2 Inflammatory diarrhea

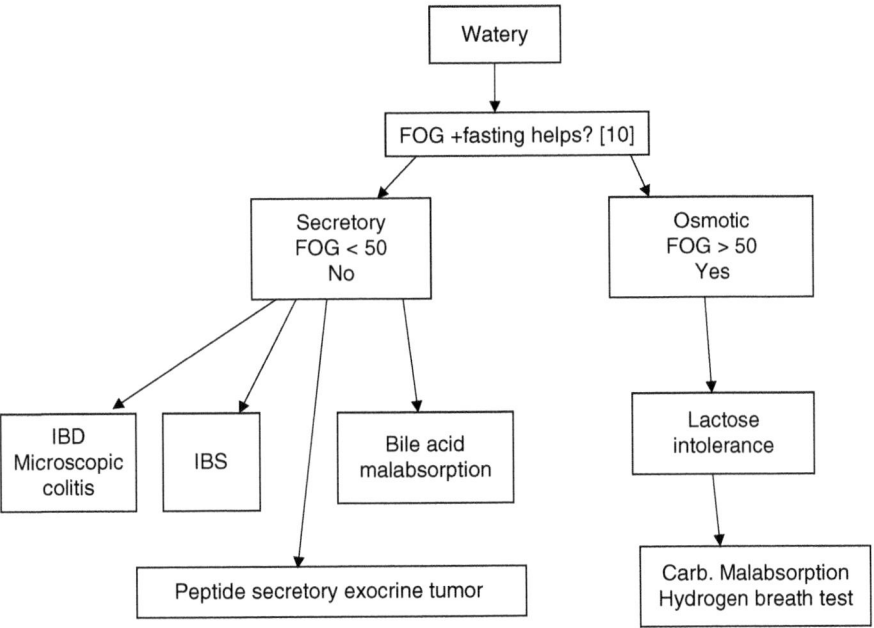

Fig. 36.3 Watery diarrhea

- Peptide secretory exocrine tumor [12]

Fecal Incontinence

- Two major types: urge and passive [13]
- Urge occurs but cannot control the urge: passive occurs without warning.
- Continence is maintained not only by sphincters but by pelvic floor muscles, anal cushions, nervous system, consistency of stools and rectal reservoir.

Fig. 36.4 Sphincter muscles and puborectalis [14]

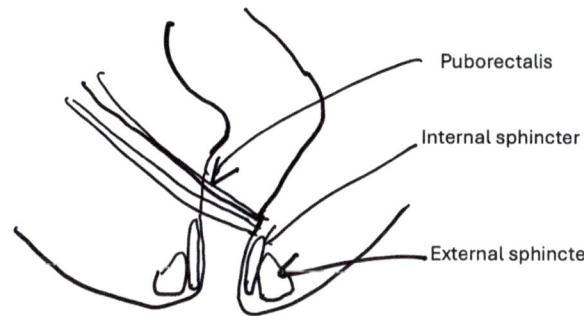

Table 36.5 Drugs exacerbate fecal incontinence

Mechanism	Drugs
Alter sphincter tone	Nitrates, calcium channel blockers, SSRI
Broad spectrum Abx	Cephalosporins, macrolides, penicillins
Topical anal drugs	Nitrate, diltiazem gel, botox
Profuse loose stools	Laxatives, metformin, SSRI, magnesium containing meds, digoxin
Constipating drugs	Loperamide, opioid, TCA,
Hypnotics	BZD, TCA, SSRI, antipsychotics

Ahmad et al. [13]

Table 36.6 Treatment

Cause	Intervention
Overflow	Disimpaction
	Scheduled defecation
Decreased storage capacity	Low fiber diet
	Loperamide
	Scheduled defecation
Sphincter weakness	Loperamide
	Anal plug
Sphincter disruption	Loperamide
Peripheral neuropathy	Sacral nerve stimulation
Dementia	Scheduled defecation/disimpaction

Wald [14]

References

1. Thielman N, Guerrant R. Acute infectious diarrhea. N Engl J Med. 2004;350:38–47.
2. Meisenheimer E, et al. Acute diarrhea in adults. Am Fam Physician. 2022;106(1):72–80.
3. ☺DuPont H. Persistent diarrhea. A clincal review. JAMA. 2016;315(24):2712–23.
4. ☺ ☺ ☺Carollo A, Schiller L. Chronic diarrhea: differential diagnosis and initial management. Consultant. 2005;45(14):1604–14.
5. Kapoor R, et al. Needle in a haystack. N Engl J Med. 2009;360:616–21.
6. Burgers K, et al. Chronic diarrhea in adults: evaluation and differential diagnosis. Am Fam Physician. 2020;101(8):472–80.
7. Arasaradnam R, et al. Guidelines for the investigation of chronic diarrhea in adults: British Society of Gastroenterology, 3rd edition. Gut. 2018;67:1380–99.
8. ☺Juckett G, Trivedi R. Evaluation of chronic diarrhea. Am Fam Physician. 2011;84(10):1119–26.
9. Schiller L, et al. Chronic diarrhea: diagnosis and management. Clin Gastroenterol Hepatol. 2017;15:182–93.
10. Binder J. Causes of chronic diarrhea. N Engl J Med. 2006;355:236–9.
11. ☺ ☺Money M, Camilleri M. Review: Management of postprandial diarrhea syndrome. Am J Med. 2012;125:538–44.
12. ☺ ☺ ☺Sweetser S. Evaluating the patients with diarrhea: a case-based approach. Mayo Clin Proc. 2012;87(6):596–602.
13. Ahmad M, et al. Management of faecal incontinence in adults. BMJ. 2010;334:1350–5.
14. ☺ ☺ ☺Wald A. Fecal incontinence in adults. N Engl J Med. 2007;356:1648–55.

Liver Cirrhosis (LC)

37

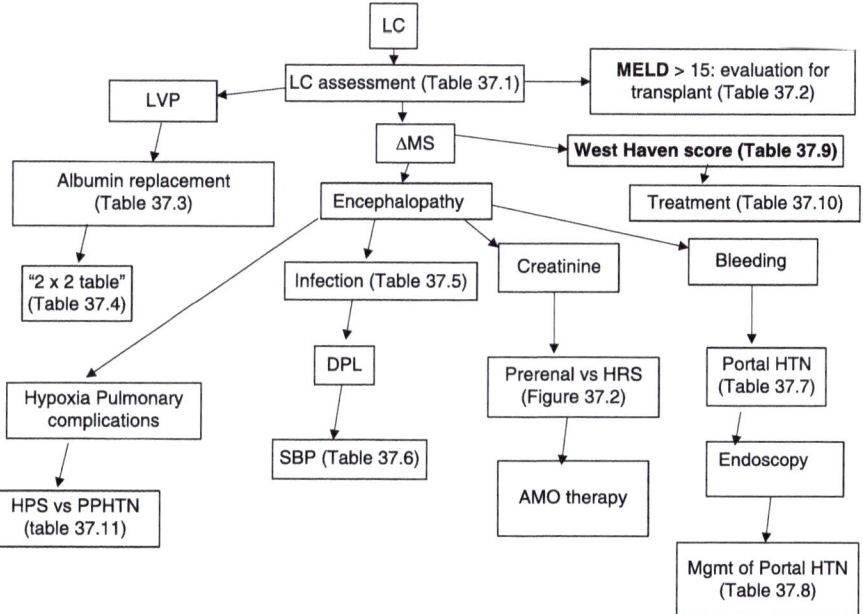

Fig. 37.1 Big picture

FACTS:

- Compensated LC has ×4.7 risk of death, decompensated LC ×9.7 [1].
- Dx of ascites, 15% die <1 year, 44% <5 years

M. J. Morikawa, *The Inpatient Medicine Handbook*,
https://doi.org/10.1007/978-3-032-08398-2_37

Table 37.1 LC assessment

- Ascites analysis is part of the vital signs:
  1. Infection: **Ascites analysis**
  2. Fluid status: **Renal/Circulatory function**
  3. Nutrition and protein synthesis ability (sarcopenia): **Liver function**

MELD > 15: evaluated for transplant [2–4]

Table 37.2 MELD score and 90-day mortality

MELD score	Mortality (%)
≤9	5.0
10–19	18.8
20–29	56.9
30–39	68.3
≥40	100

Large Volume Paracentesis (LVP)

- Refractory ascites (RA): recur after LVP despite sodium restriction and diuretic therapy

Table 37.3 Albumin replacement

Alb infusion after LVP: 8 g of Alb/L of ascites aspiration after 5 L

Biggins et al. [5]; Ge and Runyon [1]

Table 37.4 Ascites Interpretation 2 × 2 table

	SAAG < 1.1 g/dL	SAAG > 1.1 g/dL
TP < 2.5 g/dL	Nephrotic syndrome	LC
TP > 2.5 g/dL	Peritoneal disease (malignancy, TB)	RHF
		Budd-Chiari (postsinusoidal)

Biggins et al. [5]; Heidelbaugh and Sherbondy [6]

Infection

- Cirrhosis-associated immune deficiency (CAID) is the spectrum from chronic inflammation to the development of immunodeficiency [7, 8]
- PNA occurs in up to 20% of hospitalized LC patients and has a 90-day mortality of almost 35%
- Iron homeostasis affects phagocytosis and bacteriostasis, LC due to hemochromatosis are especially high risk for invasive organism, such as Vibrio vulnificus and Yersinia species [7]
- Cefotaxime is recommended as first line for SBP: ceftriaxone is more strongly protein bound than cefotaxime and hypoalbuminemic state is a concern for its effectiveness [7]

Table 37.5 LC and infection

LC + AKI or HE = R/O occult infection

Table 37.6 SBP

• Positive if one of the following:
Ascites WBC > 1000, PMN > 250, pH < 7.35 or blood-ascites pH gradient ≥0.10

Wong et al. [9]

- Once treated for SBP, repeat paracentesis at 48 h to confirm PMN decreased by 25% [8]
- When SBP + and Creatinine > 1 mg/dL, BUN > 30 mg/dL, or total bilirubin >4 mg/dL then give 1.5 g/kg of albumin <6 h with another 1 g/kg in day 3 [1]
- If ascites protein <1.5 g/dL, then oral cipro 750 mg/weekly, oral norfloxacin 400 mg/daily [10]

Portal HTN and VARICES

- Varices are present in almost 50% of patients with LC at the time of diagnosis [11]
- Gastric varices are present in 20% of patients with LC and bleeding from it is more sever and have higher mortality [11]
- The 1-year rate of recurrent variceal hemorrhage is approximately 60% [11]
- The incidence of portal vein thrombosis is approximately 16%/year in advanced LC
- Splanchnic vasoconstrictors are used in acute setting

Table 37.7 Portal HTN

Description	HVPG	Strategy
Portal HTN	≥5 mmHg	Statins?
Clinically significant	>10	Non-selective β-blocker
Increased risk of bleeding	≥12	β-blocker
		Endoscopy for banding
		Consider TIPS

Tsochatzis et al. [12]

- Stop Beta-blocker when SBP < 90 mmHg, Na < 120, or AKI [1]

Table 37.8 Agents for acute variceal bleeding

Category	Medication	Dose	Duration
Vasoconstrictor	Octreotide	50 μg bolus, 50 μg/h DIV	2–5 days
Abx	Ceftriaxone	1 g IV qd	5–7 days or until discharge
	Norfloxacin	400 mg POD BID	
Endoscopy	Ligation/sclerotherapy	Once	–

Encephalopathy

- Ammonia homeostasis is a multiple organ process and sarcopenia is associated with HE

Table 37.9 West Haven score

Grade	Feature	Hepatic encephalopathy (HE)
0	Normal	
1	Personality change, agitation	Covert HE
2	Behavioral change, cognitive dysfunction	Overt HE
3	Somnolence, confusion	
4	Coma	

Leise et al. [13]; Wijdicks [4]

Table 37.10 Treatment for HE

	Gut	Liver	Kidney	Muscle
First line tx	Lactulose/ rifaximin		Maintain euvolemia, eukalemia	Nutritional support
Second line tx	Probiotics	Zinc supplementation TIPS revision	Glycerol phenylbutyrate L-ornithine L-aspartate (LOLA)	BCAA

Tapper et al. [14]

- First episode HE: start Lacturose, ensure stool output, add rifaximin if no optimal respone [13]
- Recurrent HE: if breakthrough HE with lactulose, add rifaximin, if taking rifaximin, add lactulose. If breakthrough with lactulose + rifaximin, evaluate TIPS or consider TIPS, consider to add zinc, LOLA [13]

Severe HE (West Haven Grade 3 or 4):

1. Lactulose via NG
2. Refractory HE with MELD <12–15: look for large portosystemic shunt: if shunt+, embolization, if not shunt, add zinc, LOLA, BCAA, if no improvement, MARS (molecular absorbent recirculating system) [13]

Coagulopathy

- Conventional measures of coagulation, PT, PTT, INR doesn't assess risk of bleeding or thrombosis in advanced LC patients [15]
- Parallel reduction of procoagulants and anticoagulants coexist [16]
- FFP cannot meaningfully correct PTT in LC [17]

Pulmonary Complication

Table 37.11 Pulmonary complications

Hepatopulmonary syndrome (HPS)	Portopulmonary HTN (PPHTN)
Pulm **vasodilatation**	Pulm vasoconstriction
Hypoxia: severe	Not as bad as HPS
Orthodeoxia	Form of secondary pulm HTN only in 2–8% of LC patient
PaO2 < 50 mmHg, brain update >20% in scan is poor prognosis	PaCO2 < 30 mmHg is sensitive indicator for PPHTN

Rodriguez and Krowka [18]; Bauer et al. [19]; Budhiraja and Hassoun [20]

Renal Complication

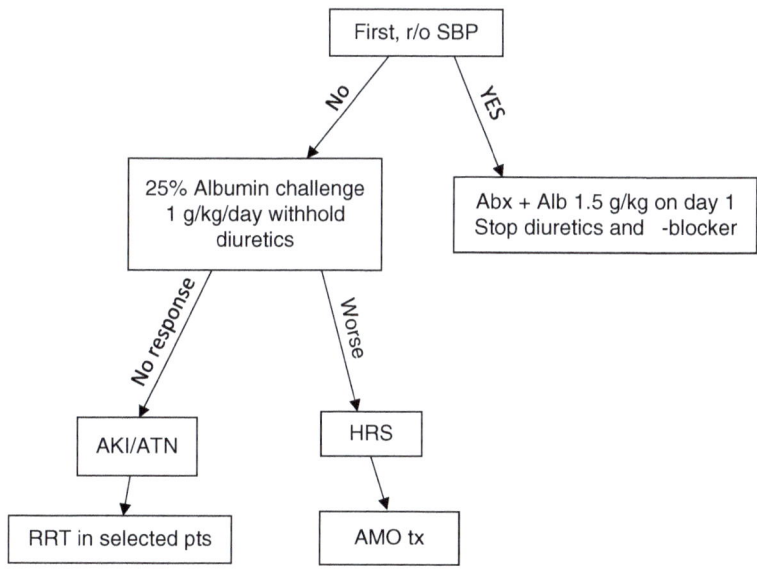

Fig. 37.2 Hepato-renal syndrome (HRS) vs AKI [21, 22]

References

1. ☺ Ge P, Runyon B. Treatment of patients with cirrhosis. N Engl J Med. 2016;375:767–77.
2. Kamath P, et al. A model to predict survival in patients with end-stage liver disease. Hepatology. 2001;33:464–70.
3. Starr S, Raines D. Cirrhosis: diagnosis, management, and prevention. Am Fam Physician. 2011;84(12):1353–9.

4. ☺☺Wijdicks E. Hepatic encephalopathy. N Engl J Med. 2016;375:1660–70.
5. Biggins S, et al. Diagnosis, evaluation, and management of ascites, spontaneous bacterial peritonitis and hepatorenal syndrome: 2021 practice guidance by the American Association for the Study of Liver Disease. Hepatology. 2021;74(2):1014–48.
6. Heidelbaugh J, Sherbondy M. Cirrhosis and chronic liver failure: Part II. Complications and treatment. Am Fam Physician. 2006;74:767–76.
7. Campbell K, et al. Infections in cirrhosis: a guide for the clinician. Am J Med. 2021;134:727–34.
8. ☺☺Bajaj J, et al. The evolving challenges of infections in cirrhosis. N Engl J Med. 2021;384:2317–30.
9. Wong C, et al. Does this patient have bacterial peritonitis or portal hypertension? How do I perform a paracentesis and analyze the results? JAMA. 2008;299:1166–78.
10. ☺Gines P, Cardenas A. Management of cirrhosis and ascites. N Engl J Med. 2004;350:1646–54.
11. Garcia-Tsao G, Bosch J. Management of varices and variceal hemorrhage in cirrhosis. N Engl J Med. 2010;362:823–32.
12. Tsochatzis E, et al. Liver cirrhosis. Lancet. 2014;383:1749–61.
13. Leise M, et al. Management of hepatic encephalopathy in the hospital. Mayo Clin Proc. 2014;89(2):241–53.
14. ☺☺Tapper E, et al. Refining the ammonia hypothesis: a physiology-driven approach to the treatment of hepatic encephalopathy. Mayo Clin Proc. 2015;90(5):646–58.
15. Allison M, et al. Hematological issues in liver disease. Crit Care Clin. 2016;32:385–96.
16. ☺Tripodi A, Mannucci P. The coagulopathy of chronic liver disease. N Engl J Med. 2011;365:147–56.
17. Dasher K, Trotter J. Intensive care unit management of liver-related coagulation disorders. Crit Care Clin. 2012;28:389–98.
18. ☺☺☺Rodriguez-Roisin R, Krowka M. Hepatopulmonary syndrome-a liver-induced lung vascular disorder. N Engl J Med. 2008;358:2378–87.
19. Bauer M, et al. Pulmonary complications in liver disease. Intensive Care Med. 2019;45:1433–5.
20. Budhiraja R, Hassoun P. Portopulmonary hypertension. A tale of two circulations. Chest. 2003;123:562–76.
21. ☺☺☺Nadim M, Garcia-Tsao G. Acute kidney injury in patients with cirrhosis. N Engl J Med. 2023;388:733–45.
22. ☺Tapper E, et al. Preventing and treating acute kidney injury among hospitalized patients with cirrhosis: a narrative review. Am J Med. 2016;129:461–7.

Dizziness

38

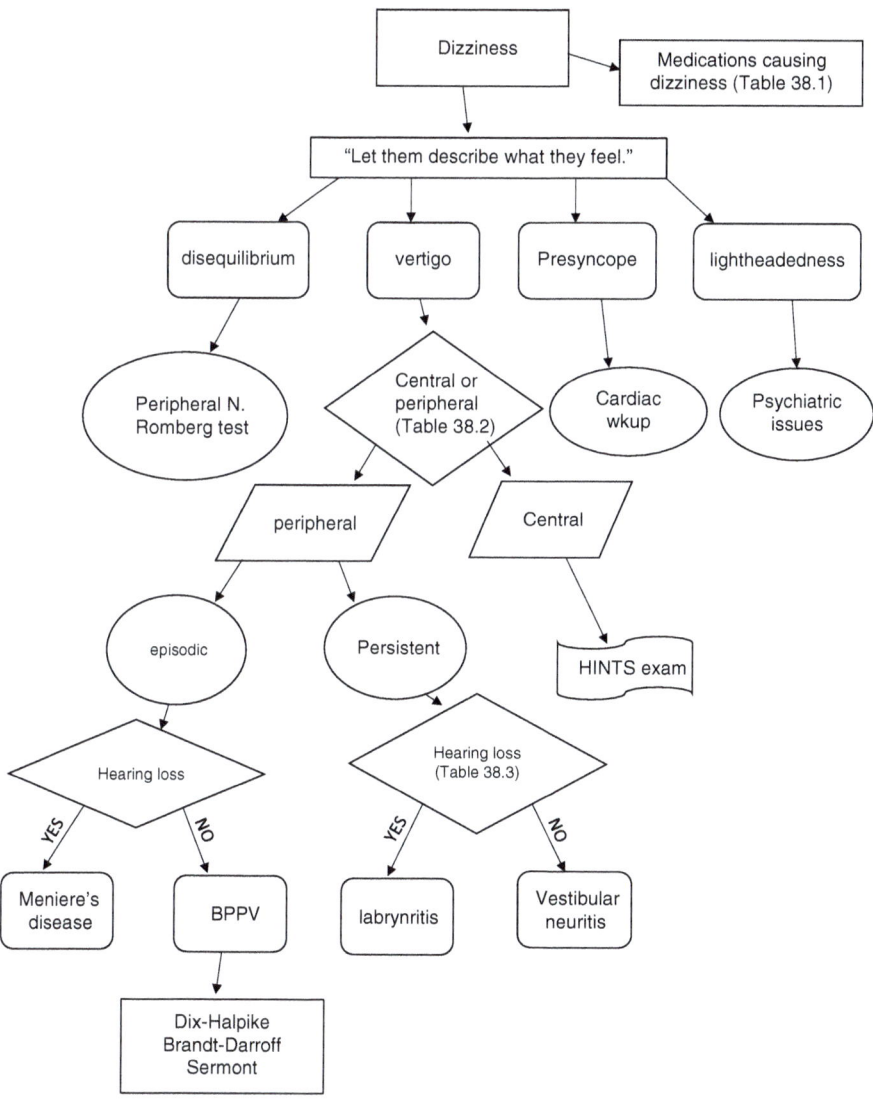

Modified from Rogers [10]; Post and Dickerson [1]; Kentala and Rauch [2]

M. J. Morikawa, *The Inpatient Medicine Handbook*,
https://doi.org/10.1007/978-3-032-08398-2_38

Table 38.1 Medications causing dizziness

\- Medications cause 23% of dizziness in primary care	
Mechanism	Medications
Cardiac effect (hypotension, OH, arrhythmias)	Alcohol, antiarrhythmics, antiepileptics, antihistamines, antihypertensives, antiparkinson narcotics, nitrates
Central anticholinergics	Muscle relaxants Antispasmodics
Cerebellar toxicity	Antiepileptics BZDs Lithium
Hypoglycemia	Antidiabetic Beta adrenergic blockers
Ototoxicity	Aminoglycosides Antirheumatic agents
Bleeding complications, BM suppression	Anticoagulants, antithyroid meds

Muncie et al. [3]

Table 38.2 Peripheral vs central vertigo

	Peripheral	Central
HIT	+	−
Stand up	+	Unable
Nystagmus	Horizontal in one direction	Changes direction with changes in the position of the gaze
Onset	Sudden	Gradual
Duration	Seconds to minutes	Weeks to months
Positional	Yes	No
Fatigable	Yes	No

Chawla and Olshaker [4]; Baloh [5]

BPPV

- Supine roll test for horizontal canal vertigo [6]

Central Dizziness

- The most common presenting symptoms of posterior circulation stroke is dizziness [7]
  HINTS exam [8]

    INFARCT: impulse normal, fast-phase alternating and re-fixation on cover test

Table 38.3 Three-parameters to categorize vertigo

		True vertigo	
		Episodic	Persistent
Hearing loss	−	BPPV	Vestibular neuritis
	+	Meniere's disease	Labyrinthitis

Kentala and Rauch [9]

References

1. Post R, Dickerson L. Dizziness: a diagnostic approach. Am Fam Physician. 2010;82(4):361–8.
2. ☺☺☺Kentala E, Rauch S. A practical assessment algorithm for diagnosis of dizziness. Otolaryngol Head Neck Surg. 2003;128:54–9.
3. Muncie H, et al. Dizziness: approach to evaluation and management. Am Fam Physician. 2017;95(3):154–62.
4. Chawla N, Olshaker J. Diagnosis and management of dizziness and vertigo. Med Clin North Am. 2006;90:291–304.
5. ☺Baloh R. Vestibular neuritis. N Engl J Med. 2003;348:1027–32.
6. ☺Huh Y, Kim J. Bedside evaluation of dizzy patients. J Clin Neurol. 2013;9(4):203–13.
7. Banerjee G, et al. Posterior circulation ischemic stroke. BMJ. 2018;361:k1185. https://doi.org/10.1136/bmj.k1185.
8. Newman-Toker D, et al. HINTS outperforms ABCD2 to screen for stroke in acute continuous vertigo and dizziness. Acad Emerg Med. 2013;20:987–96.
9. Kentala E, Rauch S. A practical assessment algorithm for diagnosis of dizziness. Otolaryngol Head Neck Surg. 2003;128:54–9.
10. Rogers TS, Noel MA, Garcia B. "Dizziness: Evaluation and management" Am Fam Physician 2023;107:514–523.

Syncope

39

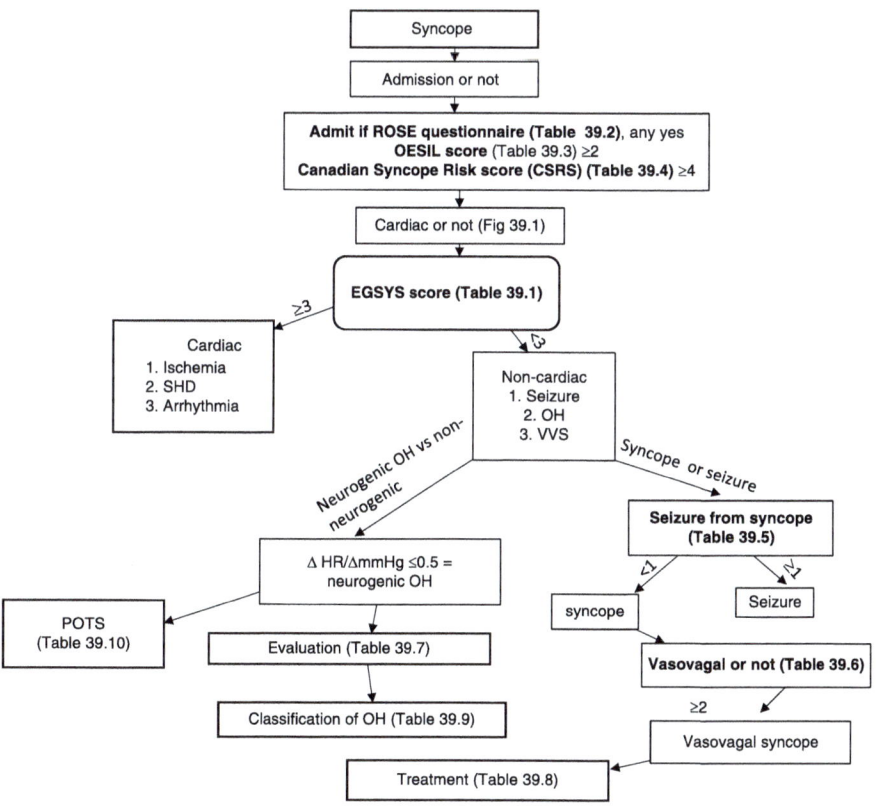

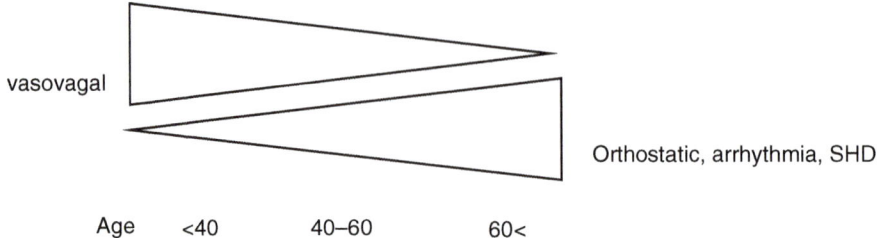

Fig. 39.1 Causes of syncope by age [1]

- The '5Ps' for hx: Precipitants; prodrome; palpitations; position; and post-event phenomena

Table 39.1 EGSYS score

Variable	Point
• The score ≥ 3 = cardiac	
Palpitation preceding syncope	4
Heart disease or abnormal EKG, or both	3
Syncope during effort	3
Syncope while supine	2
Precipitating or predisposing factors, or both (warm-crowded place/prolonged orthostasis/fear-pain-emotion)	−1
Autonomic prodromes (nausea/vomiting)	−1

EGSYS score and probability of cardiac syncope (%)	
Score	Probability (%)
<3	2
3	13
4	33
4<	77

Albassam et al. [2]; Del Rosso et al. [3]

There are several scoring system, but don't confuse general risk stratification and specific scoring to differentiate specific conditions.

General risk stratification: OESIL score, ROSE, SEEDS.

Table 39.2 OESIL score

Age >65
Hx of cardiovascular disease
Syncope without prodromes
Abnormal EKG

- The score ≥ 2 should be admitted

OESIL risk score and 12-month all-cause mortality

OESIL score	Mortality (%)
1	0.6
2	14.0
3	29.0
4	52.9

Colivicchi et al. [4]

Table 39.3 ROSE rule

• Admit any of the following are present	
• "BRACES"	
B	BNP ≥ 300 pg/mL
	Bradycardia ≤50 in ED or pre-hospital
R	Rectal exam showing fecal occult blood (GI bleeding susp)
A	Anemia Hb ≤ 9.0 g/dL
C	Chest pain associated with syncope
E	EKG showing Q wave (not in lead III)
S	Pox ≤94% on RA

Reed et al. [5]

Table 39.4 Canadian Syncope Risk Score (CSRS)

Variable	Points
Clinical evaluation	
Predisposition to vasovagal symptoms	−1
Hx of heart disease	1
SBP <90 or >180 mmHg	2
Investigations	
Elevated troponin level	2
Abnormal QRS axis	1
QRS duration >130 ms	1
Corrected QT interval >480 ms	2
Dx in ED	
Vasovagal syncope	−2
Cardiac syncope	2

Risk stratification and outcome		
Risk category	Points	Outcome (%)
Very low	<−1	0.2
Low	−1 or 0	0.7
Medium	1–3	8.0
High	4–5	19.2
Very high	5<	51.3

Thiruganasambandamoorthy et al. [6]

Table 39.5 Seizure from syncope

Variable	Point
Waking with cut tongue	2
Abnormal behavior noted	1
LOC with emotional stress	1
Postictal confusion	1
Head turning to one side during LOC	1
Prodromal déjà vu or jamais vu	1
Any presyncope	−2
LOC with prolonged standing or sitting	−2
Diaphoresis before a spell	−2

Sheldon et al. [7]

- Syncope if score <1
- Seizure if score ≥1
- Age >65, the value of the symptoms decreases [8]

Table 39.6 Vasovagal syncope or not

Variable	Point
Hx of at least one of bifascicular block, asystole, SVT, DM?	−5
Bystanders noted you turned blue during your faint?	−4
Syncope started at 35 years of age or older?	−3
Do you remember anything about being unconscious?	−2
Had lightheaded spells or faint with prolonged sitting or standing?	1
Sweat or feel warm before a faint?	2
Lightheaded spells or faint with pain or in medical setting?	3

Sheldon et al. [9]

- Vasovagal syncope if score ≥ −2

Table 39.7 Evaluation

Neurogenic OH	Autonomic evaluation
Reflex syncope	Tilt-table exam
Cardiac syncope	1. Cardiac monitor
	2. TTE, EPS, stress test

Shen et al. [10]

Table 39.8 VVS treatment

First choice	Counter pressure maneuvers
	Salt and fluid intake
Second choice	Midodrine
Third choice	Fludrocortisone
	Beta-blocker
	SSRI
	DDD pacer

Shen et al. [10]

OH Strategy

- Definition: SBP >20 mmHg or DBP >10 mmHg during the first 3 min of standing or tilt table [11]
- Nearly 50% of patients with OH have supine HTN [11], don't throw in anti-HTNs for elderly staying in the bed all day since that will make OH worse (See Chap. 24)
- Four categories of OH [12]

Table 39.9 Classification of OH

Primary neurogenic	The Alpha-synucleinopathies [13] (Table 39.2)
	PD
	LwBD
	PAF (pure autonomic failure)
	Multiple systemic atrophy (MSA)
Secondary neurogenic	Peripheral neuropathy
	DM
	EtOH
	HIV/AIDS
	Guillain0Barre syndrome
	Vit B12 def
	Spinal cord problems
Secondary non-neurogenic	Hypovolemia
	Cardiac pump failure
	Venous pooling
Drug	Vasodilators
	Diuretics
	Narcotics
	Tricyclic antidepressants
	Phenothiazines
	MAO inhibitors

Shen et al. [10]

- Schellong test and Δ HR/Δ mmHg <0.5 Neurogenic OH (Norcliffe-Kaufmann [17])
- Treatment approach for neurogenic OH similar to VVS tx above [13]

POTS:

- One of the most common chronic orthostatic intolerance [14]
- HR > 30/min within 10 min of standing without OH [15]
- Definition [16]
- Dependent acrocyanosis in leg in nearly 50% of POTS patients [16]

Table 39.10 Criteria for POTS

HR increase ≥30 from spine to standing (10 min)
Symptoms worsen with standing and improved with recumbence
Symptoms last ≥6 months
Absence of other overt causes of orthostatic symptoms or tachycardia (such as active bleeding, acute dehydration, medications)

References

1. Perry J, et al. High risk clinical characteristics for subarachnoid haemorrhage in patients with acute headache: prospective cohort study. BMJ. 2010;341:c5204. https://doi.org/10.1136/bmj.c5204.
2. Albassam O, et al. Did this patient have cardiac syncope? The rational clinical examination systematic review. JAMA. 2019;321:2448–57.
3. Del Rosso A, et al. Clinical predictors of cardiac syncope at initial evaluation in patients referred urgently to a general hospital: the EGSYS score. Heart. 2008;94:1620–6.
4. Colivicchi F, et al. Development and prospective validation of a risk stratification system for patients with syncope in the emergency department: the OESIL risk score. Eur Heart J. 2003;24:811–9.
5. Reed M, et al. The ROSE (Risk Stratification of Syncope in the Emergency Department) study. J Am Coll Cardiol. 2010;55:713–21.
6. ☺Thiruganasambandamoorthy V, et al. Multicenter emergency department validation of the Canadian syncope risk score. JAMA Intern Med. 2020;180(5):737–44.
7. ☺Sheldon R, et al. Historical criteria that distinguish syncope from seizures. J Am Coll Cardiol. 2002;40(1):142–8.
8. Del Rosso A, et al. Relation of clinical presentation of syncope to the age of patients. Am J Cardiol. 2005;96:1431–5.
9. ☺Sheldon R, et al. Diagnostic criteria for vasovagal syncope based on a quantitative history. Eur Heart J. 2006;27:344–50.
10. Shen W, et al. 2017 ACC/AHA/HRS guideline for the evaluation and management of patients with syncope. Circulation. 2017;136:e60–e122.
11. ☺☺☺Freeman R. Neurogenic orthostatic hypotension. N Engl J Med. 2008;358:615–24.

12. Goldstein D, Sharabi Y. Neurogenic orthostatic hypotension: a pathophysiological approach. Circulation. 2009;119:139–46.
13. Freeman R, et al. Orthostatic hypotension. J Am Coll Cardiol. 2018;72(11):1294–309.
14. Garland E, et al. The hemodynamic and neurohumoral phenotype of postural tachycardia syndrome. Neurology. 2007;69:790–8.
15. Benarroch E. Postural tachycardia syndrome: a heterogeneous and multifactorial disorder. Mayo Clin Proc. 2012;87(12):1214–25.
16. Raj S. Postural tachycardia syndrome (POTS). Circulation. 2013;127:2336–42.
17. Norcliffe-Kaufmann L, Kaufmann H, Palma JA, et al. "Orthostatic heart rate change in patients with autonomic failure caused by neurodegenerative synucleinopathies" Ann Neurol. 2018;83:522–31

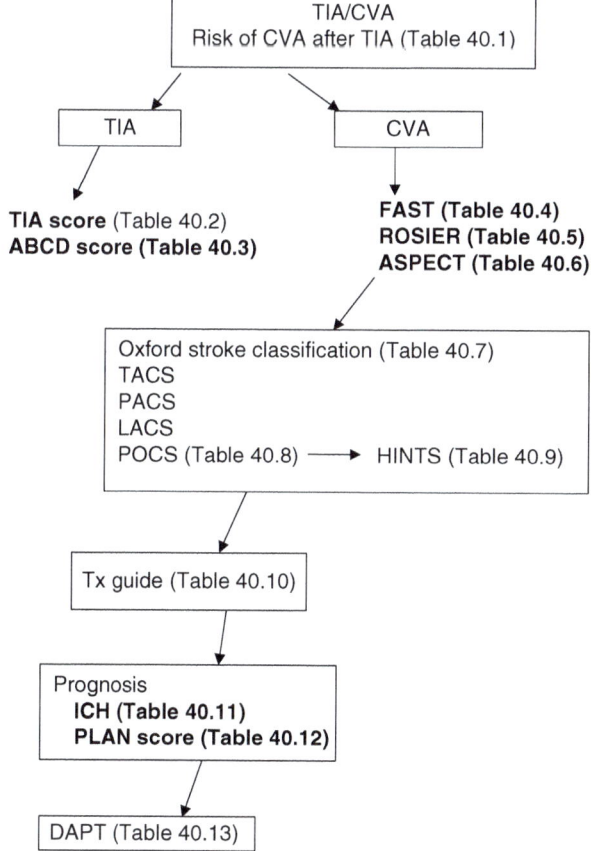

M. J. Morikawa, *The Inpatient Medicine Handbook*,

https://doi.org/10.1007/978-3-032-08398-2_40

FACTS:

TIA

- About 20–25% of patients with ischemic stroke have TIA [1]
- 10.5% of TIA presented in ED had CVA < 3 months, 5% of them had <48 h from TIA [2]
- TIA is now tissue-based diagnosis [1]

Table 40.1 Risk of subsequent stroke after TIA

Time frame	Event rate (%)
<1 year	5.9
<5 year	12.8
<10 year	19.8

Writing Committee for the PERSIST Collaborators [3]

POCS

- More than 1/3 of posterior circulation strokes are missed in the ED [4]

Cryptogenic Stroke

- Cryptogenic stroke accounts for 10–40% of all strokes [5]

ICH

- 1-year survival is 40%, 10-year is 24% [6]

TIA Scale

Table 40.2 TIA score

• Score > 6.1 (PPV 82%) or >5.4 (NPV 78%)		
Variable	Score if Yes	Score if No
Hx of CVA/TIA	0.5	0
HA	0	0.5
Diplopia	1.2	0
LOC/pre-syncope	0	1.1
Seizure	0	1.6
Speech abnormalities	1.3	0
Unilateral limb weakness	1.7	0
UMN facial weakness	0.6	0
Age	X0.04	

Dawson et al. [7]

When TIA is confirmed, risk stratify TIA for stroke risk, based on ABCD2 score [8].

Table 40.3 ABCD2 score

Variable	Points
Age ≥60	1
BP	
SBP ≥ 140 mmHg or DBP ≥ 90 mmHg	1
Clinical presentation	
Unilateral weakness	2
Speech impairment without weakness	1
DM	1
Duration of TIA	
≥60 min	2
10–59 min	1

Simmons et al. [9]

• 2-day risk of CVA from TIA based on the score

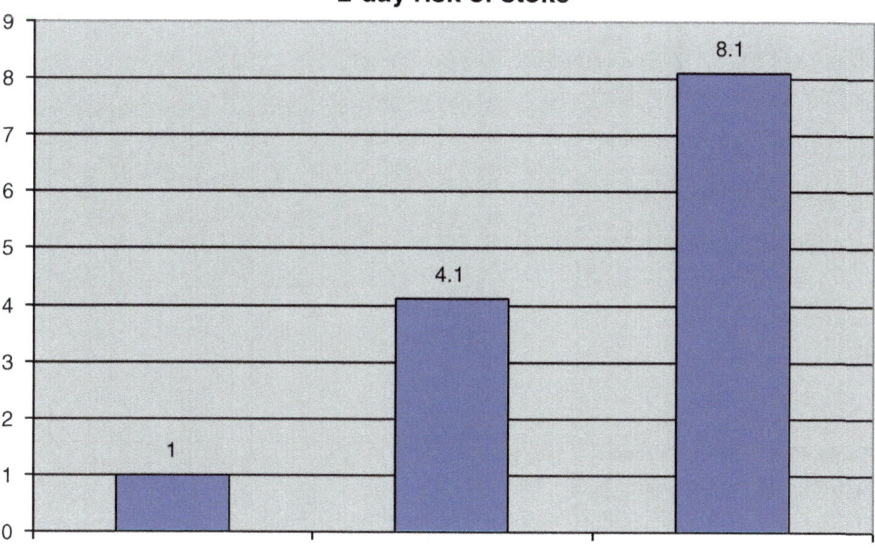

CVA Scale

Table 40.4 FAST scale

Face Arm and Speech Test (FAST)
   Face: ask the person to smile. One side of the face droop?
   Arms: ask the person to raise both arms. One arm drift downward?
   Speech: ask the person to repeat a simple phase. Speech slurred or strange?
   Time: if you observe any of the above, call 911 for ambulance

Hankey and Blacker [10]

Table 40.5 ROSIER scale

• Score > 0 and no presence of hypoglycemia, sensitivity of 92%, specificity 86%, PPV 88%, NPV 91% for stroke		
Variable	Points	
LOC or syncope	Y (−1)	N (0)
Seizure	Y (−1)	N (0)
Is there a NEW ACUTE onset (or awakening from sleep)		
Asymmetric facial weakness	Y (+1)	N (0)
Asymmetric arm weakness	Y (+1)	N (0)
Asymmetric leg weakness	Y (+1)	N (0)
Speech disturbance	Y (+1)	N (0)
Visual field defect	Y (+1)	N (0)

Nor et al. [11]

Table 40.6 ASPECTS score

For 3 months functional outcome
• Subtract score points from 10: score of 0 means diffuse ischemia
• Subcortical structures are allotted 3 points (C, L, and IC), MCA cortex is allotted 7 points (insular cortex, M1, M2, M3, M4, M5 and M6)

Feske [12]; Barber et al. [13]

Table 40.7 Oxford system of stroke classification

Classification	Symptoms

TACS (total anterior circulation stroke)	All three of the following:
	    Contralateral motor or sensory deficit
	    Homonymous hemianopia
	    Higher cortical dysfunction (includes dysphasia/ visuospatial disturbance)

PACS (partial anterior circulation stroke)	Two of the above

POCS (posterior circulation stroke)	Any one of
	    Isolated homonymous hemianopia
	    Brain stem signs
	    Cerebellar ataxia

LACS (lacunar stroke)	Any one of
	    Pure motor deficit
	    Pure sensory deficit
	    Sensorimotor deficit

McArthur [17]

Table 40.8 Posterior circulation ischemic stroke

• Common symptoms of POCS
Dizziness
Unilateral limb weakness
Dysarthria
HA
N/V

Table 40.9 HINTS exam

Horizontal **h**ead **i**mpulse test (h-**HIT**): normal
Multidirectional **n**ystagmus
Skew deviation

Banerjee et al. [4]

Table 40.10 Treatment guideline

	CVA			TIA	
	0–4.5 h	4.5–9 h	9–24 h	0–24 h	
Alteplase	+	−	−	ABCD2 < 1 MRI/CT −	ABCD2 ≥ 2 or MRI/CT +
Large vessel occlusion	Positive Endovascular tx	Positive Consider endovascular tx		N/A	NA
Antiplatelet	Negative ASA	Negative ASA but some cases (DWI + FLAIR −) consider Alteplase	Negative ASA	ASA	DAPT ×21 days then ASA

Mendelson and Prabhakaran [14]

Table 40.11 ICH risk score

Variable	Points
GCS	
3–4	2
5–12	1
13–15	0
Age	
≥80	1
<80	0
Infratentorial hemorrhage	
Yes	1
No	0
Volume (mL)	
≥30	1
<30	0
IVH	
Yes	1
No	0

Outcome	
Score	Mortality (%)
0	0
1	13
2	26
3	72
4	97
5	100

Gross et al. [6]

Table 40.12 PLAN score

• 30-day mortality	
Variable	Points
Preadmission comorbidities	
Preadmission dependence	1.5
Cancer	1.5
CHF	1
A fib	1
Level of consciousness	
Reduced	5
Age	1 point per decade
Neurological deficit	
Arm weakness	2
Leg weakness	2
Neglect or aphasia	1

30-day and 1-year mortality based on scores		
Score	30-day (%)	1-year (%)
<6	0.7	2.1
6–9	2.5	7.5
10–12	7.1	20.6
13–15	21.0	39.0
16–19	44.9	64.0
19<	65.9	83.6

O'Donnell et al. [15]

Table 40.13 Antiplatelet therapy after TIA/CVA

- DAPT (ASA + clopidogrel) started <24 h in patients with high-risk TIA (ABCD ≥ 3) or minor stroke, continue up to 21 days then should continue with single antiplatelet therapy
- DAPT is not recommended for major stoke because of the increased risk of intracranial bleeding in these patients.

Prasad et al. [16]

References

1. ☺ ☺ ☺ Amarenco P. Transient ischemic attack. N Engl J Med. 2020;382:1933–41.
2. Johnston S, Gress D. Short-term prognosis after emergency department diagnosis of TIA. JAMA. 2000;284:2901–6.
3. ☺ ☺ Writing Committee for the PERSIST Collaborators. Long-term risk of stroke after transient ischemic attack or minor stroke. JAMA. 2025;333(17):1508–19.
4. Banerjee G, et al. Posterior circulation ischemic stroke. BMJ. 2018;361:k1185. https://doi.org/10.1136/bmj.k1185.
5. Saver J. Cryptogenic stroke. N Engl J Med. 2016;374:2065–74.
6. Gross B, et al. Cerebral intraparenchymal hemorrhage. JAMA. 2019;321(13):1295–303.
7. Dawson J, et al. A recognition tool for transient ischaemic attack. Q J Med. 2009;102:43–9.
8. ☺ ☺ Johnston S, et al. Validation and refinement of scores to predict very early stroke risk after transient ischaemic attack. Lancet. 2007;369:283–92.
9. Simmons B, et al. Transient ischemic attack: Part I. Diagnosis and evaluation. Am Fam Physician. 2012;86(6):521–6.
10. Hankey G, Blacker D. Is it a stroke? BMJ. 2015;350:h56. https://doi.org/10.1136/bmj.h56.
11. Nor A, et al. The recognition of stroke in the emergency room (ROSIER) scale: development and validation of a stroke recognition instrument. Lancet Neurol. 2005;4:727–34.
12. Feske S. Ischemic stroke. Am J Med. 2021;134:1457–64.
13. Barber P, et al. Validity and reliability of a quantitative computed tomography score in predicting outcome of hyperacute stroke before thrombolytic therapy. Lancet. 2000;355:1670–4.
14. ☺ ☺ ☺ Mendelson S, Prabhakaran S. Diagnosis and management of transient ischemic attack and acute ischemic stroke. A review. JAMA. 2021;325(11):1088–98.
15. O'Donnell M, et al. The PLAN score. A bedside prediction rule for death and severe disability following acute ischemic stroke. Arch Intern Med. 2012;172(20):1548–56.
16. ☺ ☺ Prasad K, et al. Dual antiplatelet therapy with aspirin and clopidogrel for acute high risk transient ischemic attack and minor ischemic stroke: a clinical practice guideline. BMJ. 2018;363:k5130. https://doi.org/10.1136/bmj.k5130.
17. McArthur KS, Quinn TJ, Dawson J, Walters MR. "Diagnosis and management of transient ischaemic attack and ischaemic stroke in the acute phase." BMJ 2011;342:d1938 https://doi.org/10.1136/bmj.d1938.

Seizure/Epilepsy

41

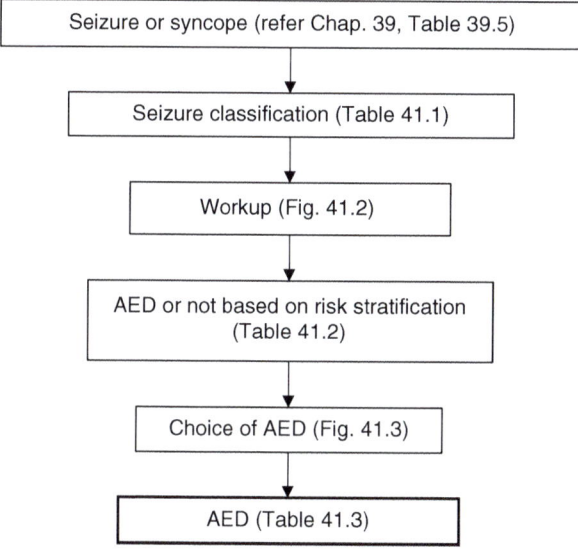

Fig. 41.1 Big picture

FACTS:

- RAMPART study (Silbergleit [7]) demonstrated IM midazolam and IV loraze-pam was equally effective for prehospital status epilepticus
- After first unprovoked seizure, the risk is the highest in first 2 years [1]
- Approx. 35% chance of recurrence in 5 years after the first seizure, but if you have a second seizure, then recurrence rate is 75% in 5 years (Gavvala [8])
- Based on MESS trial, risk score is developed [2] and the table [3] demonstrates the recurrence risk

© The Author(s), under exclusive license to Springer Nature Switzerland AG 2025
M. J. Morikawa, *The Inpatient Medicine Handbook*,
https://doi.org/10.1007/978-3-032-08398-2_41

- Immediate initiation of medicine after the first seizure had lower recurrence in the first 2 years but failed to prevent long-term seizure remission
- Krumholz consensus statement said nocturnal seizure is one of the risk factors [1]
- Low risk patient doesn't benefit from immediate treatment but potentially in medium and high-risk group
- Smith [3] made a recommendation clearer based above study

Table 41.1 Seizure classification

Nonepileptic
    1. Psychogenic nonepileptic seizure
    2. Syncope
Epileptic
    1. Provoked
    2. Unprovoked

Wilden and Cohen-Gadol [4]

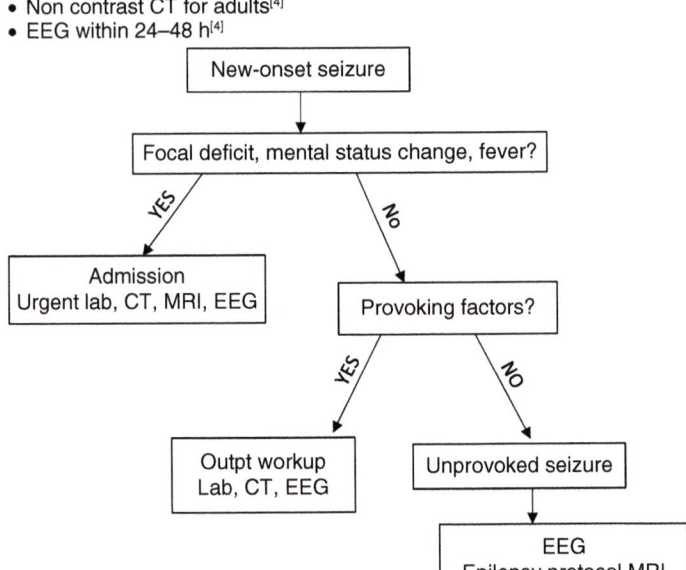

Fig. 41.2 Algorithm for workup. (Based on Gavvala (2016))

Table 41.2 Seizure risk stratification

Variable	Point
Seizures	
One seizure prior to presentation	0
2–3 seizures prior to presentation	1
≥4 seizures prior to presentation	2
Neurological findings	
Neurological disorder/deficit/learning disability or developmental delay	1
Abnormal EEG	1

Risk category and score	
Risk category	Score
Low	0
Medium	1
High	2–4

Probability of seizure by 5 years immediate tx vs delayed group			
Risk category	Immediate tx	Delayed	Meds
Low	0.39	0.30	No
Medium	0.39	0.56	Consider
High	0.50	0.73	Yes

Table 41.3 AED

Narrow-spectrum	Broad-spectrum
Carbamazepine	Lamotrigine
Gabapentin	Levetiracetam
Phenytoin	Topiramate
Eslicarbazepine	Valproate
Oxcarbazepine	Zonisamide

Gavvala (2016); Asadi-Pooya et al. [5]

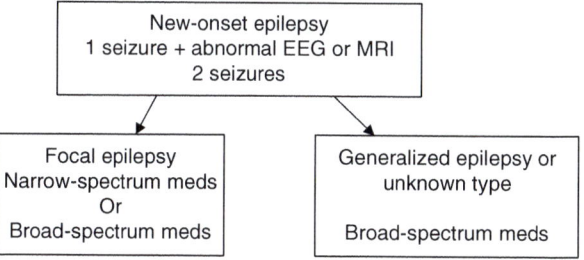

Fig. 41.3 AED choice

- For elderly, lamotrigine or gabapentin are better tolerated (Gavvala 2016)
- AED should be started as monotherapy and titrate up [6]
- Antiseizure medications are effective around 2/3 of patients [5]
- Choice of AED in the setting of comorbidities [6]
- AED for women and risk of major congenital malformation [6]

References

1. Krumholz A, et al. Evidence-based guideline: management of an unprovoked first seizure in adults. Neurology. 2015;84:1705–13.
2. ☺☺Kim L, et al. Prediction of risk of seizure recurrence after a single seizure and early epilepsy: further results from the MESS trial. Lancet Neurol. 2006;5:317–22.
3. ☺☺☺Smith P. Initial management of seizure in adults. New Engl J Med. 2021;385:251–63.
4. ☺Wilden J, Cohen-Gadol A. Evaluation of first nonfebrile seizures. Am Fam Physician. 2012;86(4):334–40.
5. ☺☺Asadi-Pooya A, et al. Adult epilepsy. Lancet. 2023;402:412–24.
6. Kanner A, Bicchi M. Antiseizure medications for adult with epilepsy. A review. JAMA. 2022;327(13):1269–81.
7. Silbergleit R, Durkalski V, Lowenstein D, et al. Intramuscular versus intravenous therapy for prehospital status epilepticus. N Engl J Med. 2012;366:591–600.
8. Gavvala JR, Schuele SU. New-onset seizure in adults and adolescents. A review. JAMA. 2016;316:2657–68.

Part IV

Essential Formula

Essential Formulas 2025

© The Author(s), under exclusive license to Springer Nature Switzerland AG 2025
M. J. Morikawa, *The Inpatient Medicine Handbook*,
https://doi.org/10.1007/978-3-032-08398-2_42

Index